# Co-Creating a Holistic Healing Environment in Nursing Practice

# Co-Creating a Holistic Healing Environment in Nursing Practice

FIRST EDITION

SHIRLEY C. GORDON AND NANCEY E.M. FRANCE
Florida Atlantic University

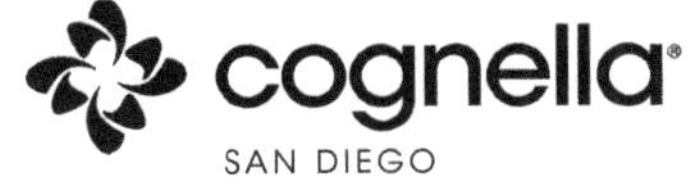
SAN DIEGO

Bassim Hamadeh, CEO and Publisher
Seidy Cruz, Specialist Acquisitions Editor
Gem Rabanera, Senior Project Editor
Casey Hands, Production Editor
Monica O'Keefe, Editorial Assistant
Jess Estrella, Senior Graphic Designer
JoHannah McDonald, Licensing Coordinator
Natalie Piccotti, Director of Marketing
Kassie Graves, Senior Vice President, Editorial
Jamie Giganti, Director of Academic Publishing



Printed in the United States of America.



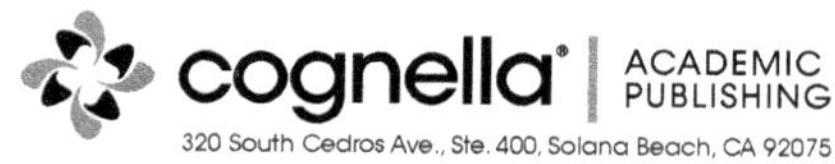

*We dedicate this book to all Nurses as they knowingly participate in changing patterns and rediscover their power as healers to co-create a holistic healing environment.*

# About the Artwork

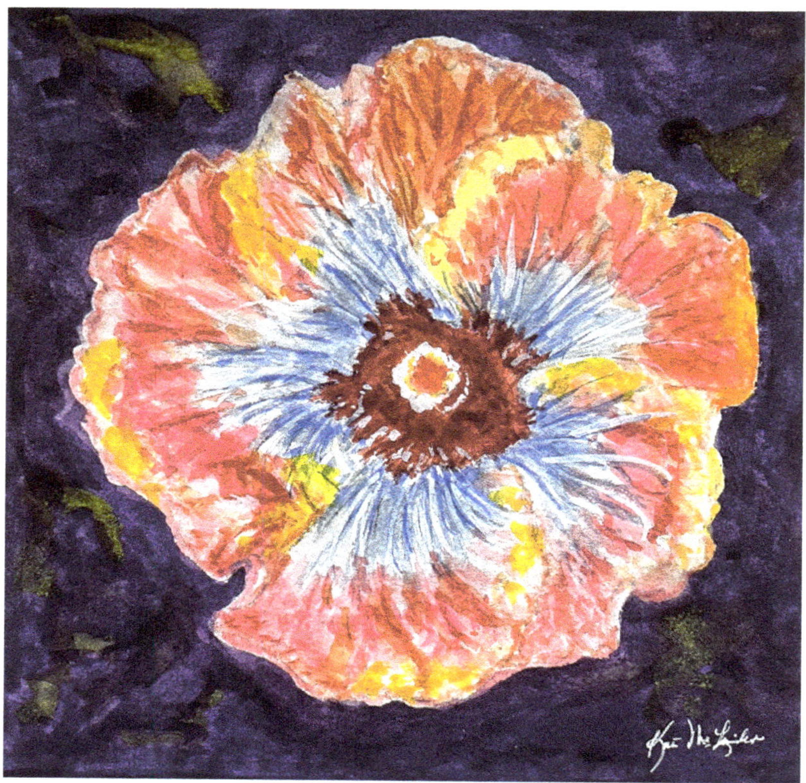

Kathleen McLinden, "Hibiscus moscheutos: Healing through and within Caring." Copyright © by Shirley C. Gordon and Nancey E.M. France. Reprinted with permission.

The essence of the Holistic Healing Environment framework is revealed within nature's *Hibiscus moscheutos*. Within its intricate design, we experience alternating rhythms and patterning in mutual process from the petals to its center symbolizing the emergence of compassionate unity and healing. The beauty and meaning of art are in the *heartmindbodysoul* of the beholder. We, therefore, entitle this divine art of nature "*healing through and within caring.*"

# Brief Contents

# Detailed Contents

## ACTIVE LEARNING

This book has interactive activities available to complement your reading.

Your instructor may have customized the selection of activities available for your unique course. Please check with your professor to verify whether your class will access this content through the Cognella Active Learning portal (http://active.cognella.com) or through your home learning management system.

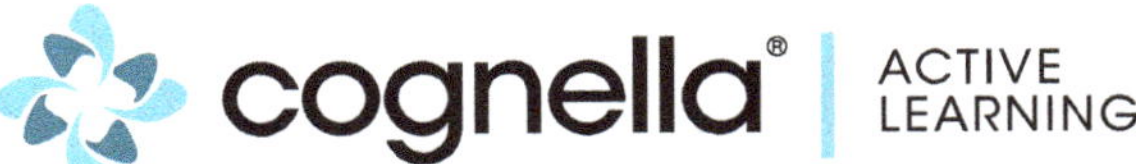


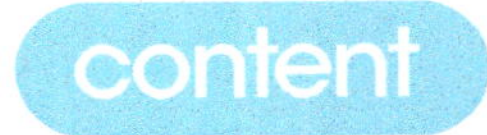

## WEB-BASED RESOURCES: ACCESSING QR CODES AND LINKS

The authors have selected some supporting web-based content for further engagement with the learning material that appears in this text, which can be accessed through QR codes or web links. These codes are intended for use by those who have purchased print copies of the book. You may scan them using a QR code reading app on your cell phone, which will take you to each website. You can also search for the link using a web browser search engine. Readers who have purchased a digital copy of the book can simply click on the hyperlinks beneath each QR code.

Cognella maintains no responsibility for the content nor availability of third-party links. However, Cognella makes every effort to keep its texts current. Broken links may be reported to studentreviews@cognella.com. Please include the book's title, author, and 7-digit SKU reference number (found below the barcode on the back cover of the book) in the body of your message.

Please check with your professor to confirm whether your class will access this content independently or collectively.

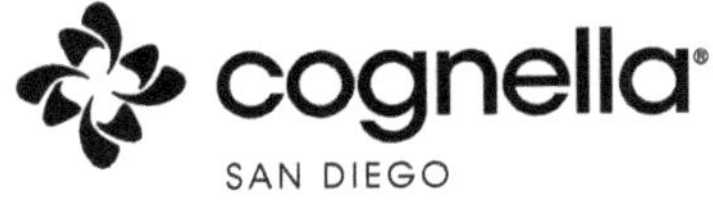

# Foreword

*Jean Watson, PhD, RN, AHN-BC, FAAN, LL (AAN)*

With so much of today's attention on the crisis of Nursing and hospitals, and a national focus on supporting and advancing the profession of Nursing, here enters this book: *Co-creating a Holistic-Healing Environment in Nursing Practice*, by Shirley Gordon and Nancey France. Here we are invited into a much deeper dimension of Nursing *qua Nursing*, rescuing and restoring the very heart and soul of Nursing; embodied through generating and initiating a holistic healing environment for self and system.

Through this original, co-creative scholarship, the reader enters into a journey, participating in living-out and codesigning a holistic healing environment; this work transcends conventional practices and mindsets yet grounds the very foundation of Nursing—past, present, future. This foundation is translated throughout the book, affirming the discipline of Nursing within the Unitary-Transformative Paradigm. The result—a more mature holistic Nursing praxis guided by a mature professional, disciplinary-specific framework.

This Unitary-Transformative framework expands and deepens the very heart and soul of Nursing and transmutes all areas of concern for its evolution, if not the survival, of Nursing as a holistic discipline. Concepts such a *Nurse as Soul Whisperer* and *Healer* are exemplars of the transmutation which occurs when holistic Nursing practice is elevated to, and located within, the unitary cosmic energy field of sacred circle of life/death, and all the in-betweens.

The invitation and opportunity evolving from within this framework is nothing short of a decoding of the historic and futuristic primary purpose and praxis of holistic Nursing. This decoding and application is transposed into concrete constructive action and directions for now and the future.

The process unfolds within the flow of the units and chapters into living design exemplars manifesting in micro and macro settings for education and practice—both actual and virtual. Likewise, in keeping with the heart and soul of the holistic framework, the closing chapters embody the history of Nursing and Nurses in war and pandemic, bringing the living history forward full circle into the pandemic of our time.

For anyone seeking to help Nursing embrace, evolve, and embody its *raison d'être* for being/becoming, here you find the invitation and 'way shower' to inspire, inform, transform, and transcend self and system. This seeking then becomes a call for sacred holistic action across time and space into a new future calling us forward.

# Introduction

Why this book at this time? Nursing is the most trusted profession in the United States (Saad, 2022). After suffering through the COVID-19 pandemic, the world witnessed first-hand the necessity and imperative for Nurses and Nursing. It is our hope this book inspires Nurses to rediscover their power and resilience as the center of healthcare—Nurse as soul whisperer and healer.

Language is powerful. In the book, we have capitalized *Nurse* and *Nursing* to honor and respect our colleagues, discipline, science, art, and profession. We encourage you and the world to continue this movement.

So, you may be asking, "how is this book different from other books?" Many of you may be familiar with and/or use the term *optimal healing environments*; however, we have come to know and understand that there are no optimal healing environments in Nursing. There is only a holistic healing environment: *Dance of alternating rhythms with intentional knowing participation to co-create an environment through which holistic healing emerges for Nurse and person(s).*

This book, deeply grounded in unitary caring science, introduces the Holistic Healing Environment (HHE) Framework, and guides the Nurse on the *why and how* of co-creating a holistic healing environment. We included key concepts at the beginning of each chapter to help the reader grasp the depth of meaning inherent in the language of the Unitary-Transformative Paradigm.

The intended audiences are:

- All academic programs of Nursing (undergraduate, masters, doctoral)
  - Student Nurses and faculty
- Professional Nurse development
  - All Nurses in any practice setting
- Anyone who seeks to know more about Nursing as a discipline, science, art, profession
  - Other healthcare providers, administrators, and researchers

Within the HHE Framework, the focus of Nursing is healing and the call for Nurse is to co-create an environment of holistic healing to transcend suffering. The purpose of the framework is to guide the Nurse in co-creating a holistic healing environment in which healing emerges within and through caring. The HHE Framework does not stand by itself but is philosophically congruent with caring theories of Nursing in the Unitary-Transformative Paradigm.

In Unit I, ***The Soul of the Holistic Healing Environment Framework,*** we present the HHE Framework and provide a foundation for understanding the Unitary-Transformative Paradigm. In this context, soul reflects the emotional/intellectual energy of the framework.

In Unit II, ***Co-Creating a Holistic Healing Environment: Nurses' Living Experiences,*** we introduce you to five expert Nurses who each co-create a holistic healing environment moment-by-moment.

Through the profound words from the Nurses' living experience, within the HHE Framework the imperative for healing within and through caring for self to care for another is revealed.

In Unit III, ***Designing Educational Experiences within the Holistic Healing Environment Framework***, we illuminate how the HHE Framework may be manifested within educational experiences. The HHE Framework is integral regardless of the educational setting.

In the final unit, Unit IV, ***Co-Creating a Holistic Healing Environment to Ease Suffering and Restore Humanness and Humanity During Times of War and Pandemic,*** we focus on the imperative to co-create a holistic healing environment within the worst of the worst conditions. Historical accounts and personal interviews with Nurses who shared their living experiences show us that as Nurses we do not get to choose those conditions, and we are called to co-create healing through and within caring moment-to-moment. For many Nurses around the world, war and/or pandemic have become everyday practice.

Each chapter is carefully constructed to challenge your thinking and begins with objectives that provide a consistent content structure followed by key concepts that provide a quick reference to understanding the chapter. Thoughtful reflections are an invitation to pause and reflect on what you have read and are intentionally designed to facilitate knowing. The Nursing Situation is integral to experiencing the essence of HHE Framework and exemplars are presented throughout the book. Vastly different from the medical case study, the Nursing Situation is the aesthetic expression of the Nurse's living experience within praxis grounded in caring science, embodies all patterns of knowing, and focuses on what matters most to persons. Suggested individual and group learning activities at the end of each chapter encourage self-reflection and exploration of the HHE Framework.

As you begin your journey of coming to know and live the HHE Framework, we invite you to immerse yourself within the patterns, rhythms, and flow of Unit I *in its wholeness* before experiencing the other chapters. In Units II, III, and IV, we explore the beauty and power of Nursing in a variety of practice settings through the lens of the HHE Framework. In the Appendix, we share the living experiences of the rich Nursing Situations embedded throughout the book as an invaluable resource for faculty and program developers. The Nursing Situations, while site- and population-specific, can be interwoven within a range of courses or professional development programs across populations and settings.

We commissioned artist Kate McLinden to create original watercolor paintings as aesthetic expressions of Nurse as soul whisperer, healing through and within caring and the HHE Framework.

> *After reconnecting with my college roommate, Dr. Nancey E. M. France, I felt honored and privileged to paint all three of the watercolors for this book, especially the painting titled Nurse as Soul Whisperer. With having my own medical issues over the years and the ongoing COVID-19 pandemic, it gave me a different perspective on the career of a Nurse. Just painting the two masks and shield on the face of the Nurse, her gloved hand reaching out to her elderly patient and perfecting her eyes intensely connecting with his, made me realize they truly are soul whisperers on a day-to-day basis. As a new artist and a communications/public relations specialist for nearly 50 years, I realized a career in Nursing must be a heart-wrenching challenge, everyday. While I have always had fabulous care from the Nurses I have encountered, I now have a more intimate, up-close and personal appreciation for all of them. (Kate McLinden, personal communication, May 13, 2022)*

It is our intention and hope that you continually grow in your understanding and come to know Nurse and Nursing in profound and exciting new ways. We welcome your responses to the HHE Framework and invite you to share Nursing Situations and living experiences of how the framework impacts your praxis with us!

Shirley C. Gordon, PhD, RN, NCSN,
AHN-BC, HWNC-BC | Professor | Director
Initiative for Intentional Health

Nancey E. M. France PhD, RN, AHN-BC,
HWNC-BC | Professor Emerita | Trauma-Sensitive
HeartMath® Certified Practitioner | Clinical
Faculty Integrative Nurse Coach Academy

# UNIT I

# The Soul of the Holistic Healing Environment Framework

## Introduction

We welcome you to Unit I as you begin the incredible journey of co-creating a holistic healing environment! This unit is of primary importance to the book in its *wholeness* and emerges from our *passion* for Nursing, grounded in our practice/teaching/learning experiences.

In Unit I, we reveal the soul of the Holistic Healing Environment (HHE) Framework. You might be wondering—how can a framework have a soul? As person and environment are an integral energy field in continuous mutual interaction, the environment is dynamic, living, always in motion. In this context, soul reflects the emotional/intellectual energy of the framework.

We encourage you to read the chapters in Unit 1 in the order they are presented. So, we begin with reviewing, perhaps for some of you redefining, *Nurse* and *Nursing*. A basic assumption of this book is that Nurse is soul whisperer and healer. Chapter 1 provides a context for understanding Nursing as a science, discipline, art, and profession grounded in the Unitary-Transformative Paradigm. Building on this understanding, Chapter 2 explores the evolution of knowledge and praxis within Nursing from which the HHE Framework emerges. In Chapter 3, the HHE Framework is presented and includes a practice exemplar of how to integrate the framework in co-creating an environment for holistic healing for Nurse and person.

Each chapter is carefully constructed to challenge your thinking. Chapter objectives, key concepts, prewriting activities and thoughtful reflections are intentionally designed to facilitate learning. It is our intention that you grow in your understanding and come to know Nurse and Nursing in a profound and exciting new way.

1

# Nurse as Soul Whisperer and Healer

*Nurse (noun): co-creator of healing and peace through caring science; helps person to find meaning in the living experience and wellbecoming; soul whisperer, healer.*

## Introduction

This chapter defines the **Nurse as soul whisperer** (a term first coined by Phillips, 2015) **and healer**, emerging from Nursing as science, discipline, art, and profession. When someone asks you, "What do you do?," is your first response, "I'm a Nurse" or "I'm in Nursing school"? When you tell someone you are a Nurse or studying to become a Nurse, rarely does the person then ask, "What is a Nurse, and what does a Nurse do?" But, if you were asked to define "Nurse" and describe the role of a Nurse, what would you say?

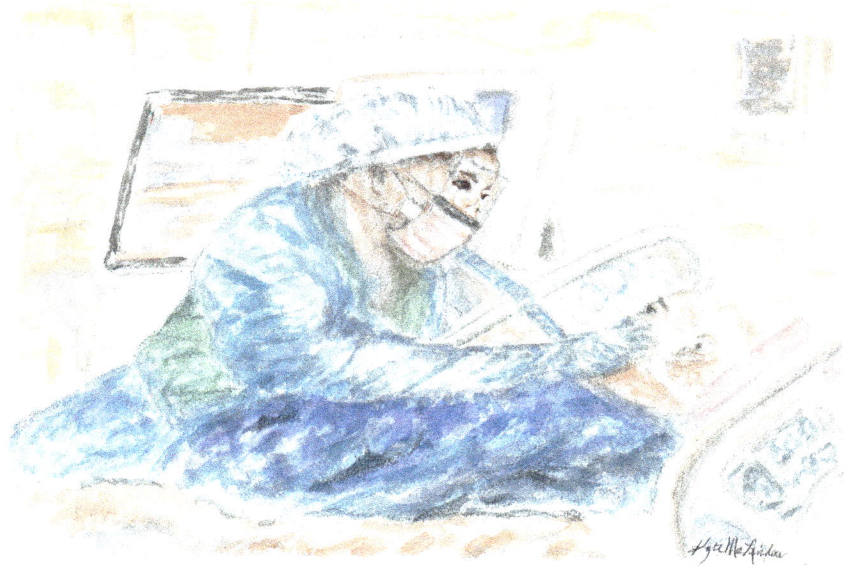

**FIGURE 1.1** Nurse as Soul Whisperer and Healer. Kathleen McLinden, "Nurse as Soul Whisperer and Healer." Copyright © by Shirley C. Gordon and Nancey E.M. France. Reprinted with permission.

Take a moment to reflect—how do you define Nurse and your role as a Nurse? And then we'll move on.

### Objectives

After completing this chapter, readers will:

1. Define
    a. Nursing as a discipline, science, and art
    b. Nursing as a profession
    c. Nursing praxis
2. Come to know the Nurse as soul whisperer and healer
3. Understand living the role of Nurse as soul whisperer and healer requires:
    a. Caring for self
    b. Being authentically present
    c. Becoming integrally present
    d. Co-experiencing compassionate unity and healing

### Key Terms and Concepts

- **Nursing**—A basic and applied science, discipline, art with its own unique, abstract, and substantive body of knowledge created from basic and applied research and development and testing of its theories; a learned profession. Persons who are educated to use Nursing knowledge (science) according to nationally regulated, defined, and monitored standards for the protection and safety of healthcare for society and its members are *Nurses.*
- **Nursing praxis**—The interconnectedness of a discipline's worldview, science, theories, research, education, and practice emerging as "a synthesis of thoughtful reflection, caring, and action within theory and research-driven practice" (Hines & Gaughan, 2014, p. 26); a synchrony of knowing/doing/being (Watson, 2018, p. 21).
- **Holistic**—Greater than and different from the sum of parts.
- **Wholeness**—*Heartmindbodysoul.*
- **Nursing profession**—Defined within praxis; "consists of persons educated in the [Nursing] discipline according to nationally regulated, defined, and monitored standards (Parse, 1999, p. 275) for the protection and safety of healthcare for society and its members.
- **Nursing Situation**—The aesthetic expression of the Nurse's living experience within praxis grounded in caring science and embodies all patterns of knowing and focuses on what matters most to persons.

- **Nurse**—*Co-creator of healing and peace through unitary caring science; helps person to find meaning in the living experience and wellbecoming; soul whisperer, healer.*
- **Soul Whisperer**—Nurse interconnects with person soul-to-soul through "pandimensional thoughts such as soothing, tender, quieting, and loving, giving illumination and radiance" (Phillips, 2015, p. 46) to transcend suffering.
- **Living experience**—Repeating and enduring energy pattern(s) of a person's past/present/future life experience.
- **Wellbecoming**—A process through which one knowingly participates in changing patterns and manifestations of wholeness and healing.
- **Caring for self**—Holistic blueprint for wholeness and self-healing through coming to know self in our wholeness and what matters most to us within our *heartmindbodysoul.*
- **Inner coherence**—The person's *heartmindbodysoul* is in harmony and synchrony.
- **Resilience**—"The *capacity to prepare* for, recover from and adapt in the face of stress, adversity, trauma, or tragedy" (HeartMath® Institute, 2021a, para 3 ln 1–2).
- **Trauma**—"The subjective experience of an event, or series of events, that overwhelms an individual's capacity to cope" (HeartMath® Institute, 2021b, p. 1).
- **Authentic presence**—Awareness of and coming-to-know self in synchrony and harmony within alternating rhythms guided by Mayeroff's ingredients of caring and Roach's caring attributes to choose *who I bring to practice in this moment.*
- **Integral presence**—"A perceiving-experiencing of the integrality of [persons] and the environment" (Phillips, 2015, p. 46) emerging from authentic presence, as the Nurse experiences the wholeness of self and other and the interconnectedness of self with other.
- **Compassionate unity**—Emerges within integral presence and is the alternating rhythms of perceiving-experiencing *I feel you, you feel me, and I feel you feeling me* (Hübl, 2021, p. 2)—the interwoven energy field of Nurse and simultaneously the healer and healee, both healing and both being healed. Within compassionate unity, Nurse is soul whisperer and healer.

## The Science and Art of Nursing

For years, many have talked about the science and art of Nursing. "Historically the term **'Nursing'** has been used as a verb signifying 'to do,' rather than as a noun meaning 'to know.' When Nursing is identified as a science the term 'Nursing' becomes a noun signifying a body of abstract knowledge" (Rogers, 1992, p. 29). Nursing has its own unique, abstract, substantive body of knowledge (science), which is created from basic and applied research and development and testing of its theories. Nurses are educated to use Nursing knowledge (science) and integrate patterns of knowing to guide their praxis. This is the art of Nursing.

Aesthetics, a pattern of knowing, is concerned with the art of Nursing. The art of Nursing is "the imaginative and creative use of knowledge" (Rogers, 1988, p. 100) and emerges as an aesthetic expression of knowing and pattern appreciation in practice. Therefore, the science and art of Nursing are lived within the Nurse as healer.

## Nursing as a Discipline

While most people acknowledge Nursing as a profession, many do not understand that Nursing is first a discipline, a science, and an art. A discipline has its own unique substantive body of knowledge that "provides a means of describing and explaining the discipline's phenomena of central concern" (Rogers, 1992, p. 28). Within the discipline's unique substantive body of knowledge are theories. Theory is generally understood as an abstract notion showing relationships between and among concepts and phenomena.

> Theories deriving from a science of unitary human beings are specific to Nursing, just as theories deriving from biology are specific to biological phenomena, theories deriving from sociology are specific to sociological phenomena, and theories deriving from physics are specific to the physical world. The study of Nursing is not the study of the biological world any more than the study of biology is the study of the physical world. Further, the study of Nursing is not the study of Nurses and what they do any more than the study of biology is of biologists and what they do. Nursing instead, is the study of unitary, irreducible, indivisible human and environmental fields: people and their world. (Rogers, 1992, p. 29)

"The goal of the [Nursing] discipline is to expand knowledge about human experiences through creative conceptualization and research" (Parse, 1999, p. 275). This knowledge creates the science that guides living the art of Nursing (Parse, 1999). Nursing science is understood as both a basic and an applied science. As a basic science, Nurse researchers explore what it means *to know* what is unique to Nursing with caring as the essence of Nursing (Boykin & Schoenhofer, 2001). As an applied science, Nurse researchers seek to understand what it means *to do* in the practice of Nursing.

While Florence Nightingale was the first to identify Nursing as a science and an art, Jean Watson was the first to elevate "the concept of caring into the realm of hard science" (University of Colorado Anschutz Medical Campus (2013) by uniting "quantum thinking of Rogers's science with caring science" (Watson, 2020, p. 313). Watson also focused the discipline's phenomena of central concern on "human caring, healing, and health" (Watson, 2020, p. 313).

The discipline's phenomena of central concern and unique focus are based on the theoretical framework used by the Nurse to guide practice. For example, Nightingale's first assumption is "Nursing is separate from medicine" (Dunphy 2020, p. 48). For Watson, "[Nursing] science has a meaningful philosophical foundation, a value foundation about humanity. It's not about medical treatment and cure. [Nursing] is not a subset of medicine" (Watson Caring Science Institute, 2017).

Martha Rogers (1992) more clearly defines the phenomena central to Nursing's purpose as "indivisible human and environmental energy fields" (Society of Rogerian Scholars, n.d.-b); however, these phenomena are often reduced to *person, environment, health* as have been described by Nightingale and others throughout Nursing's history. Watson's caritas processes evolved from the mutual process of the human and environment energy fields and "provide a voice and a language for the phenomena of Nursing," which makes them visible (Watson Caring Science Institute, 2017) revealing the power of Nurse as healer.

## Nursing as a Profession

Nursing is "a learned profession" (Rogers, 1992, p. 28). The Nursing profession "consists of persons educated in the discipline according to nationally regulated, defined, and monitored standards" (Parse, 1999, p. 275) for the protection and safety of healthcare for society and its members. Regulations and standards are designed and enforced by agencies such as the American Nurses Association (ANA) (Social Policy Statement, Standards of Practice, Code of Ethics), National Council of State Boards of Nursing (NCSBN), American Association of Colleges of Nursing (AACN), Commission on Collegiate Nursing Education (CCNE), and Accreditation Commission for Education in Nursing (ACEN). Persons educated within the discipline of Nursing and who are licensed as professional Nurses can practice following national and state Nursing regulations and Nursing standards.

As professionals, Nurses may choose to belong to professional Nursing organizations to specialize in an area of Nursing practice and seek certification. Licensure and certification acknowledge this expertise and assure society of quality, safe healthcare.

"Although the discipline and the profession of nursing have different goals, the raison d'être of nursing is the enhancement of quality of life for humankind. The discipline provides the science lived in the art of practice" (Parse, 1999, p. 275).

## The Call to Nursing

At the beginning of the chapter, you were asked how you would respond to the question "What do you do." After answering, "I'm a Nurse"' or "I'm in Nursing school," the next question is often "Why?" or "How did you know you wanted to be a Nurse?" This section offers insights into the call to Nursing experienced by three Nurse theorists whose work guides our understanding of Nurse as soul whisperer and healer: Nightingale, Rogers, and Watson. Additionally, you are encouraged to read the primary works and contemporary interpretations of the theorists.

### Florence Nightingale

Nightingale was born into in a wealthy aristocratic family. She was the younger of two daughters, both of whom are named after cities in Italy—Florence and Parthenope—and were well educated by their father in a time when society did not value the education of women. Mr. Nightingale provided his daughters with a classical Cambridge home education, which included "music; grammar; composition; modern languages; classical Greek and Latin; constitutional history; Roman, Italian, German and Turkish history; and mathematics" (Dunphy, 2020, p. 37). The Nightingales traveled with their daughters to France, Italy, Switzerland, Egypt, and Greece (Dunphy, 2020, p. 37).

Around the age of 17, Nightingale experienced a "calling from God" to serve humanity. On her own, Nightingale traveled to Germany where she learned about a Protestant religious community in Kaiserswerth that provided training to women "who wished to nurse" (Dunphy, 2020, p. 37).

Even though Nightingale's family did not permit her to be a Nurse, as those women were considered to be of ill-repute, she returned to and enrolled in Nurses training at Kaiserswerth. After Nurses training, she traveled to Ireland "touring hospitals and keeping notes on various institutions" (Dunphy, 2020, p. 37). Then she traveled to Paris where she took more hospital training and accepted her "first official Nursing post as superintendent of an Establishment for Gentle Women in Distressed Circumstances during Illness" (Dunphy, 2020, p. 37). Nightingale left her position as superintendent when she was appointed by Britain's minister of war to practice in a war zone. She was charged with leading Nurses to care for wounded and sick soldiers during the Crimean War.

Nightingale was the first Nurse theorist, expert researcher, and statistician, who forced her way onto multidisciplinary teams, demanded and instituted evidence-based healthcare and healthcare reform, served an environmental activist, and advocated for human rights and social justice especially for women and children (Dossey, 2021, personal communication). Nightingale developed and introduced policies to protect vulnerable persons and populations and designed and elevated Nursing education and the role of the Nurse to "support the environment to assist the patient in healing" (Dunphy, 2020, p. 48).

Nightingale spent over 23 years practicing and preparing herself and others for what was to become modern Nursing, which she founded in 1860 at the age of 40. Many describe her as a rebel, a visionary, and a healer.

## Martha E. Rogers

Four years following the death of Nightingale, Martha Rogers was born on May 12, 1914—the same birthday as Nightingale (May 12, 1820). Interestingly, when asked when she started conceptualizing the Science of Unitary Human Beings, Rogers stated, "I started when I was born" (cited in Hektor, 1994b, p. 18).

Rogers was the oldest of four children (Malinski, 1994). She loved books; when she was old enough to read, she would check out eight books at a time from the public library. "By the fourth grade, I had read every book in the school library" (Hektor, 1994a, p. 13).

As Rogers completed high school and not sure exactly what she wanted to do, she entered the University of Tennessee at Knoxville. She knew she wanted to help people, so she considered law and medicine. After two years, still struggling with wanting to help people and to do something, Rogers chose Nursing. "It was really serendipitous that I got into Nursing. I knew nothing about Nursing when I decided to become a nurse" (Hektor, 1994a, p. 13). Her parents, however, viewed Nursing as an undesirable field, believing that a liberal arts education or home economics "were good fields for women" (Hektor, 1994a, p. 13).

Rogers entered the Knoxville General Hospital Nursing School and left after a few weeks. She shared:

> The discipline was Army, pre-Nightingale. You had to stand up for everyone; it really wasn't for me. I left, went home, spent a miserable week. I remember riding the bus one day to the end of the line, looking at all the tired people—working class people, you know, so I went back to Nursing school. (cited in Hektor, 1994a, p. 14)

She described Nursing school as "full of surprises and challenges," caring for persons from different lifestyles, with different languages and social values (Hektor, 1994a, p. 14). As there was no library at the school, in her determination she started one.

Upon completion of her Nurses training, Rogers then attended George Peabody College in Nashville to not only "please her parents" to earn a college degree but also for "her own need for continued intellectual stimulation and growth" (Hektor, 1994a, p. 14). She earned a Bachelor of Science degree in public health Nursing and started her Nursing career as a public health Nurse in rural Michigan.

After two years practicing in Michigan, Rogers went on to school to earn a Master of Public Health degree at Teacher's College at Columbia University. While going to school, she practiced as a public health Nurse at the Visiting Nurse Association.

While at the Visiting Nurse Association, she "was assigned to a district with 66 different nationalities" (Hektor, 1994b, p. 16). "We exercised freedom and autonomy. We were responsible for our own acts. We were never accountable to other disciplines" (cited in Hektor, 1994b, p. 16). Rogers loved being a public health Nurse. "What I liked was seeing people where they were in their homes, and the promotion of health" (cited in Hektor, 1994b, p. 15). After she graduated with her master's degree, Rogers moved to Phoenix to start the Visiting Nurse Service and served as its executive director.

Rogers left Arizona for Johns Hopkins University to pursue her doctorate. In 1954, Rogers was appointed the head of the Division of Nursing at New York University. She revised the curriculum to increase substantive Nursing knowledge and research in Nursing focusing on people. In her 1966 address to Nursing students at New York University, Rogers stated:

> Nursing's story is a magnificent epic of service to [humankind]. It is about people: how they are born, and live and die; in health and in sickness; in joy and in sorrow. Its mission is the translation of knowledge into human service. Nursing is compassionate concern for human beings. It is the heart that understands and the hand that soothes. It is the intellect that synthesizes many learnings into meaningful administrations. (Society of Rogerian Scholars, n.d.-a)

In 1970, Rogers published her work introducing what would later be named the Science of Unitary Human Beings in the 1980s. Like Nightingale, Rogers had a "passionate love for nursing. [She] was consistent, some would say persistent, and determined in her love for nursing" (Phillips, 2015, p. 43). "Rogers was forthright, sometimes blunt, in her advocacy for nursing as a science and an art" (Phillips, 2015, p. 44). Rogers laid the foundation for Nurse as healer when she called for autonomous

Nursing practice and noninvasive healing modalities. As Rogers was blazing the trail for Nursing, Watson was beginning her own journey as Nurse healer.

## Jean Watson

Watson is the youngest of eight children and remembers paying attention "to what was going on around me in terms of all the human dimensions and complexities of life and suffering" (Watson Caring Science Institute, 2017). "My father died very suddenly when I was 16 years old and I think that influenced me ... in terms of dealing with loss and grief ... That inspired me when I went into Nursing school because I was sensitive to people and their suffering (Watson Caring Science Institute, 2017).

Watson entered the diploma program at the Lewis-Gale School of Nursing. She states, "I critiqued Nursing school because it was always about medicine, ... diagnoses, disease, ... pathology, ... treatment, ... cure, ... procedures and tests ... and following the rules so to speak" (Watson Science Institute, 2017). She continues, "There was never any attention to the human dimensions of our caring and what we were actually doing. ... There was never any philosophical conceptual information to grasp the complexities of our humanity" (Watson Science Institute, 2017). The relationships she had with her patients were very meaningful, personal, and rewarding to her.

Watson started her Nursing career in psychiatric Nursing at a large state hospital outside Baltimore that also included a very progressive research center. In this practice, Watson describes how she felt encouraged:

> ... to have that human-to-human connection of authenticity [with patients] ... [to connect] with their feelings and who they were behind their diagnoses. ... That was a very meaningful, personal experience for me because I felt I was connecting with people and their subjective life world ... I was intrigued by the mystery and knowing of what was behind their suffering ... their pain, ... their distress; what was happening to their spiritual life in their heart so to speak. (Watson Caring Science Institute, 2017)

During this time of psychiatric Nursing practice, Watson became aware of a Nurse who was getting her doctorate at Boston College.

> I was so inspired because I didn't ever know it was possible to get a doctorate in Nursing at that time. It was very rare—there were only two or three in the country. And so, I secretly said to myself that's what I want to do. (Watson Caring Science Institute, 2017)

Watson continued her education earning a Bachelor of Science in Nursing, then a Master of Science in psychiatric mental-health Nursing with a minor in psychology, and then a PhD in educational psychology and counseling. When she finished her PhD, she joined the faculty at the University of Colorado, which she describes as a "mixed experience"—"it was a very progressive curriculum ... but the faculty were still wanting to advance Nursing qua medicine under medical science" (Watson Caring Science Institute, 2017). In 1979 Watson wrote her first book, *Nursing: The Philosophy and Science of Caring,* identifying the caritive factors that were the core of Nursing—the essentials of human caring transcending variables such as setting, diagnosis, location, age.

Watson herself kept evolving as did her ideas and her theory. She then transposed the caritive factors to the ten caritas processes. The word *caritas* was chosen as it brings "more meaning to human caring and love and healing and health and energy, compassion" (Watson Caring Science Institute, 2021a).

She then developed a model of caring science—more explicit beyond medicine and the Western worldview of science, which she states "separates us rather than unites us" (Watson Caring Science Institute, 2017). Watson clearly differentiates Nursing science from medical science. For Watson, Nurses practicing within Unitary Caring Science are part of a healing model that is congruent with Nurse as healer.

**Thoughtful Reflection**

So, now, take a moment and ask yourself—what is my call to Nursing? Why am I a Nurse? Why am I in Nursing school? How did I *know*?

## The Emergence of Nurse as Soul Whisperer and Healer

> *The power in the Nurse's healing is often hidden in the subtle compassionate actions such as spending extra time with a patient or a family in crisis or the subtle effect of compassionate and calming words and the gentle touch of soothing hands* (Butcher, 2021, para 16).

The phenomenon of Nurse as soul whisperer and healer emerges from an understanding of Nursing as a discipline and a profession. The Nurse as soul whisperer and healer can be understood and studied through the use of Nursing Situations (Barry, Gordon, & King, 2015). A Nursing Situation is the aesthetic expression of the Nurse's living experience within praxis grounded in caring science, embodies all patterns of knowing, and focuses on what matters most to persons. A Nursing Situation is different from a case study. A case study is grounded in the medical model and focuses on the pattern of empirical knowing including objective and subjective data. The following Nursing Situation, written from the perspective of the Nurse, captures the essence of Nurse as soul whisperer and healer as depicted in Figure 1.1.

## Nursing Situation: "I'm Your Nurse. And I'm Here with You"

*It's Sunday and my first 12-hour shift of the week. I work on a COVID unit. I have two patients assigned to me already, both on ventilators and I'm getting my third. The Emergency Department Nurse called and gave me report—81-year-old white male, overweight, mild CHF, hypertension, shortness of breath, cough, Temp 100.9, COVID positive. States no ventilator. I gather the team asking how everyone is this morning—we don PPE and begin getting the room ready. We welcome the respiratory therapist as he arrives with BPAP equipment. The elevator doors open, and the ED team brings in our patient.*

*I can see that he's struggling to breathe. We rush him into the room, transfer and position him, calibrate alarms, connect monitors, check lines, start BPAP. As a team we work in synchrony, trusting each person's competence. With the technology and team communication, there's so much noise. I give the team-approved hand signal to now lower the human noise in this environment. The respiratory therapist shifts his position so I can get as close as possible to our patient given the restrictions of PPE.*

*I lean down, touch his bare shoulder, still being able to feel the clamminess of his skin with my gloved hand. "Mr. W" looks at me, our eyes connecting us in this moment. I see fear in his eyes. I am deeply aware that my eyes, my touch, my energy must co-create a healing environment for him in this chaos. Within this moment, we are integrally present and in compassionate unity. "I'm Susan, your Nurse. And I'm here with you." I see a tear escape his left eye and run down his cheek.* (France & Gordon, 2021)

Envisioning the Nurse as healer is not a new phenomenon. Nightingale stated, "It will take 150 years for the world to see the kind of Nursing I envision" (cited in Dossey & Luck, 2015, p. 389).

Nightingale's vision and mission were to promote healing for persons and their environment through disease prevention and health promotion. Nightingale had a holistic approach to healthcare clearly stating that the Nurse was "to create the conditions that best promoted healing" (McDonald, 2013, p. 36 https://cwfn.uoguelph.ca/short-papers-excerpts/the-timeless-wisdom-of-florence-nightingale/), making visible the "power in the Nurse's healing" (Butcher, 2021, para 16 https://pressbooks.uiowa.edu/rogeriannursingscience/chapter/chapter-5-introduction-to-the-principles/).

More recently, Watson stated that "work provides a distinct focus for the discipline of Nursing for caring and healing ..." (2018, p. xix). Watson describes caring science as sacred science and uses the "word caritas to bring meaning to human caring, love, and healing" (Watson Caring Science Institute, 2017). Rogers (1992) also addressed healing and Nursing when she called for Nurses to have autonomy in practice to provide community-based health services and noninvasive therapeutic healing modalities such as therapeutic touch, imagery, meditation, color, sound, motion, and humor.

Let's revisit the definition of Nurse from the beginning of this chapter to explore how the Nurse *becomes* the co-creator of healing and peace, helping persons, families, and communities find meaning in the living experience and wellbecoming.

> *Nurse (noun): co-creator of healing and peace through unitary caring science; helps persons, families, communities find meaning in the living experience and wellbecoming; soul whisperer, healer.*

The term, wellbecoming, first coined by Phillips (2015), is uniquely defined within the Holistic Healing Environment (HHE) Framework as a process through which one knowingly participates in changing patterns and manifestations of wholeness and healing.

*Nurse as soul whisperer and healer* starts with the Nurse holistically caring for self as energyspirit following Mayeroff's (1971) ingredients of caring—knowing, alternating rhythms, patience, honesty, trust, humility, hope, and courage. This means having the courage, patience, and humility to be honest in coming-to-know self in alternating rhythms and having trust and hope during this daily journey. Coming-to-know is having awareness of who you choose to bring to practice in that moment.

Caring for self holistically is different from self-care. Self-care focuses on strategies to address our deficits and weaknesses—and they're often grounded in feeling guilty or being upset with ourselves. A focus on strategies provides a piece-by-piece plan trying to balance everything to fix us. Self-care strategies are often unrealistic. or we just do not have time or are too tired to follow the plan.

Caring for self holistically starts with coming to know self in our wholeness and what matters most to us within our *heartmindbodysoul*. Caring for self is grounded in healing and loving; appreciating our strengths as well as what needs to be strengthened; and forgiving our stumbles and blunders. So, caring for self is a holistic blueprint for wholeness and self-healing with integrative daily approaches that helps us strengthen our "*capacity* to *prepare* for, recover from and adapt in the face of stress, adversity, trauma, or tragedy" (HeartMath® Institute, 2021a, para 3).

Caring for self begins with awareness/mindfulness practices such as those researched by the HeartMath® Institute. HeartMath® techniques begin with heart-focused breathing that helps us to ground and center, shifting our energyspirit to inner coherence, enhancing our ability to be authentically present with ourselves and others.

Authentic presence with ourselves emerges through inner coherence when the person's *heartmindbodysoul* is in harmony and synchrony. Authentic presence requires holding that awareness within alternating rhythms guided by Roach's caring attributes: compassion, competence, comportment, conscience, confidence, and commitment (commonly referred to as the 6 *C*s).

Within authentic presence, the Nurse perceives and experiences the wholeness of self and other and the interconnectedness of self with other, known as integral presence. Integral presence, first coined by Phillips (2015), emerges from Rogers' (1992) Principle of Integrality. Within the HHE Framework, the meaning of integral presence is "a perceiving-experiencing of the integrality of [persons] and the environment ..." (Phillips, 2015, p. 46) emerging from authentic presence, as the Nurse experiences the wholeness of self and other and the interconnectedness of self with other.

Within integral presence emerges compassionate unity as the Nurse and other co-create a holistic healing environment. Compassionate unity is manifested within the alternating rhythms of perceiving-experiencing "*I feel you, you feel me, and I feel you feeling me*" (Hübl, 2021, p. 2)—the interwoven energy field of Nurse and other, simultaneously the healer and healee. Both Nurse and other experience healing and are both being healed. Within compassionate unity, Nurse is soul whisperer and healer.

Phillips (2015) suggests "a person's soul manifests an array of phenomena such as peace, joy, bliss, sense of hungering, and feelings of soul being bruised, wounded, tortured, and scarred" (p. 46) and raises the following question: "What about a soul weeping for tenderness and dignity, the quivering of the soul in the throes of physical death and unexpressed cries of the soul?" (p. 46).

Within compassionate unity, Nurse is soul whisperer and healer as she/he experiences/perceives a deeper pandimensional awareness of soul-to-soul mutual knowing to transcend suffering. The Nurse understands person in one's wholeness as energyspirit. Therefore, when the Nurse touches another's body, she/he is simultaneously touching their heart, mind, body, AND soul (*heartmindbodysoul*). Nurse interconnects with person soul-to-soul through "pandimensional thoughts such as soothing, tender, quieting, and loving, giving illumination and radiance" (Phillips, 2015, p. 46) to transcend suffering. Nurse as soul whisperer and healer within compassionate unity is a sacred manifestation of caring.

**Thoughtful Reflection**

How does the Nurse as soul whisperer and healer practice?

There is no protocol or step-by-step guide. Nurse as soul whisperer and healer is in continuous mutual process with the environment and with intention chooses to *knowingly participate.* Authentic presence, integral presence, and compassionate unity are not linear but pandimensional and emerge within and through alternating rhythms and mutual patterning. In practice, Nurse as soul whisperer and healer

- cares for self in his/her wholeness—*heartmindbodysoul*—increasing inner coherence and strengthening resilience
- before entering the practice setting, the patient's room, or a meeting, grounds and centers for awareness of and coming-to-know self in synchrony and harmony within alternating rhythms to prepare *with intention* for authentic presence, mindfully shifting to *who do I choose to bring to practice in this moment?*
    - in becoming authentically present, the Nurse "manifests fundamental respect for human dignity" (American Nurses Association, n.d., para 3) as he/she knowingly engages with the healthcare team during report, hand-off, and coming to know the other (person/patient, Nurse, family, healthcare team members)
- within the practice setting, becomes integrally present through perceiving-experiencing the integrality of Nurse and environment—the wholeness of self and the interconnectedness of self with other: the patient, members of the healthcare team, and families/significant others
    - uses critical thinking, patterns of knowing to guide holistic assessment, diagnosis, and treatment of the human response to trauma of the *heartmindbodysoul*
    - advocating for persons, families, communities, and populations for quality care in healthcare settings by knowingly participating in and pursuing policies at institutional, local, regional, state, and federal levels that assure equality, equity, and social justice
- emerges from integral presence to compassionate unity through and within the alternating rhythms of perceiving-experiencing *I feel you, you feel me, and I feel you feeling me* (Hübl, 2021, p. 2)—the interwoven energy field of Nurse and other, simultaneously the healer and healee, both healing and being healed
    - co-designs holistic Nursing care with the patient and/or significant other and/or family as she/he mindfully and critically evaluates and integrates multidisciplinary plans of care (i.e., medicine, physical therapy, respiratory therapy) to assure safe, holistic healing
    - helps person to find meaning in the living experience, transcend suffering for healing
    - practicing tirelessly to identify and protect the needs of the individual (American Nurses Association, n.d. para 1).

## Summary

This chapter defined the Nurse as soul whisperer and healer, emerging from Nursing as science (basic and applied), art, discipline, and profession. Nightingale, Rogers, and Watson were selected as the exemplars of Nurses who continue to have a significant, powerful, and meaningful impact on Nursing. Their passion for Nursing is manifested in their lifelong commitment and service for the betterment and healing of persons wherever they are—in any environment or setting—advocating for human rights and social justice. Nightingale, Rogers, and Watson clearly articulated that Nursing is separate from medicine and other disciplines, and Nurses have autonomy of practice.

Nurses are the experts in Nursing, therefore, someone who is not a licensed professional Nurse cannot direct the practice of Nursing. Nurses are *equal partners* in healthcare in any setting, exploring with the patient, family, and other members of the healthcare team to codesign strategies for healing that answer the question "What matters most to person?" Nurses are the center of the healthcare team. This does not necessarily mean the "leader." although many times Nurse is in this role. Nurses look at everything holistically and see the person in his/her wholeness; we "see" the whole in the parts and the parts in the whole to heal suffering. Nurse is soul whisperer and healer.

## Key Takeaways from This Chapter

The phenomenon of Nurse as soul whisperer and healer emerges from an understanding of Nursing as science, art, discipline, and profession. Below is a list of key information and ideas to take away from your reading.

- *Nurse* is a noun and not a verb.
- *Nursing* as a science is a noun meaning "to know," "signifying a body of abstract knowledge" (Rogers, 1992, p. 29).
- Nursing is a discipline with its own science and is not a subset of medicine.
- Nursing's science, Unitary Caring Science, is considered a basic and applied science.
- As a basic science, Nurse researchers explore what it means to know what is unique to Nursing with caring as the essence of Nursing (Boykin & Schoenhofer, 2001). As an applied science, Nurse researchers seek to understand what it means *to do* what is required in the practice of Nursing.
- Unitary Caring Science guides living the art of Nursing.
- Nursing is "a learned profession" (Rogers, 1992, p. 28). The Nursing profession "consists of persons educated in the discipline according to nationally regulated, defined, and monitored standards" (Parse, 1999, p. 275) for the protection and safety of healthcare for society and its members.

- The Nurse as soul whisperer and healer must first care for self holistically and come to know self as energyspirit in our wholeness before holistically caring for another in his/her wholeness, be grounded and centered, and authentically present to self to then become integrally present with another.

## End-of-Chapter Questions, Applications, and Group Activities

**Directions:** Use what you have learned in this chapter to reflect upon and respond to the questions and prompts below.

### Questions

- In your own words, explain
  - Nursing as a discipline, science, art, profession
  - Difference between praxis and practice
  - Why Nursing is not a subset of medicine
  - Nursing as a profession and who are members of this profession
  - Nurse as soul whisperer and healer

### Applications

- Reflect on your call to Nursing.
- Reflect on the following: How do you holistically care for self in your wholeness? How does this differ from self-care?
- Create a holistic caring-for-self plan with two or three measurable outcomes. Keep a journal on what's working well for you, and how you are feeling over the next two weeks.
- How does holistically caring for self help prepare you for authentic presence?

### Group Activities

- Write down your personal call to Nursing—don't put your name on it. Then gather and look across all the responses. Do you see any enduring repeating patterns? Does anything in particular emerge for you that you hadn't realized in yourself?
- Take a minute to read this reflection. Share your thoughts on Nurse as soul whisperer and healer.

  *Before I entered graduate school, I had never heard the terms Nurse, soul whisperer, and healer used together. I was unaware of the true meaning of Nursing and what it means to be a soul whisperer and healer. When I think back to my Nursing education and work experience, there was greater focus on disease management with very little attention on understanding the art and science of Nursing, healing, and caring for self. Through gaining this insight, I have more clarity and purpose in my personal life and work life. I am empowered to help other Nurses recognize the true healing nature within each one of us. Through self-awareness and healing, as Nurses we can evoke a paradigm shift in healthcare focused on healing the mind, body, and spirit using holistic modalities and self-care strategies.*

- Revisit the Nursing Situation *"I'm Your Nurse. And I'm Here with You"* presented in the chapter. Where are the following manifested—authentic presence, center of the team, integral presence, and compassionate unity? Give specific examples.
- How did this Nursing Situation and activity affect you? What did you come to *know*?

2

# Underpinnings of the Holistic Healing Environment Framework

## Introduction

This chapter presents the underpinnings or foundations essential to understanding the development and purpose of the Holistic Healing Environment (HHE) Framework. The underpinnings of the framework include evolution of knowledge and praxis within Nursing as a discipline; metaparadigm and phenomena central to Nursing; worldview or paradigm; and selected caring theories of Nursing. The purpose of the HHE Framework, grounded in the Unitary-Transformative (UT) Paradigm, is to guide the Nurse in concert with caring theories of Nursing in co-creating a holistic healing environment within and through caring.

**Objectives**

After completing this chapter, readers will:

1. Describe the evolution of knowledge and praxis within Nursing as a Discipline.
2. Define phenomena central to Nursing.
3. Identify examples of caring theories of Nursing within the Unitary-Transformative Paradigm.

**Key Terms and Concepts**

- **Person**—A person is understood as an energyspirit (Phillips, 2015), which is "an irreducible, indivisible, pandimensional energy field identified by pattern and manifesting characteristics that are specific to the whole and which cannot be predicted from knowledge of the parts" (Rogers, 1992, p. 29). The concepts person and energyspirit are used interchangeably throughout the book.
- **Environment**—Environment is understood as "an irreducible, pandimensional energy field identified by pattern and is integral with the human field" (Rogers, 1992, p. 29).

The person-environment field includes everything external to and interacting with person (energyspirit) in a continuous mutual process.

- **Health**—Within the Unitary-Transformative Paradigm and HHE Framework, wellbecoming replaces the static concepts of health and wellbeing.
- **Nurse**—*Co-creator of healing and peace through unitary caring science; helps person to find meaning in the living experience and wellbecoming; soul whisperer, healer.*
- **Praxis**—The interconnectedness of a discipline's worldview, science, theories, research, education, and practice emerging as "a synthesis of thoughtful reflection, caring, and action within theory and research-driven practice" (Hines & Gaughan, 2014, p. 26); a synchrony of knowing/doing/being (Watson, 2018, p. 21).
- **Pandimensionality**—A "nonlinear domain without spatial or temporal attributes" (Rogers, 1992, p. 29).
- **Wellbecoming**—A process through which one knowingly participates in changing patterns and manifestations of wholeness and healing.
- **Intention**—The choice to knowingly participate in the person-environment field.
- **Knowing participation**—The intentional mutual patterning within person and environment, which are unitary and inseparable.
- **Energyspirit**—Replaces the concepts of person or patient and "unifies energy and spirit as a whole and transcends ideas of parts, including mind-body-spirit" (Phillips, 2017, p. 223).
- **Living experience**—Repeating and enduring energy pattern(s) of a person's past/present/future life experience.

## Metaparadigm, Worldview, and Phenomena Central to Nursing

As a discipline of knowledge, Nursing defines its practice by identifying a set of concepts known as a metaparadigm. A metaparadigm is the domain of inquiry or focus of a discipline and provides the foundation of the knowledge structure for any discipline (Smith & Parker, 2020, p. 11). The metaparadigm of Nursing consists of four concepts or phenomena of interest: person, environment, health, and Nurse. From the metaparadigm emerges the worldview, also known as a paradigm, that "encompasses a coherent, interrelated set of basic beliefs about the phenomena of concern" (Cody, 1995, p. 144) and from which a discipline's science, theories, research, education, and practice arise and create/design the discipline's science/knowledge.

Disciplines do not share the same metaparadigm and paradigm; therefore, their science/knowledge consists of different values or beliefs, phenomena of concern, and theories—for example, medicine's metaparadigm and paradigm are different from Nursing's metaparadigm and paradigm because they are two distinct disciplines.

The metaparadigm, paradigm, science, and theories must be in synchrony—all interconnecting with shared meaning to guide research, education, and practice, which then flow back supporting the theory, science, paradigm, and metaparadigm. This synchrony represents the evolution of praxis, which is the discipline and profession in its *wholeness*. Figure 2.1 demonstrates the evolution of praxis within Nursing.

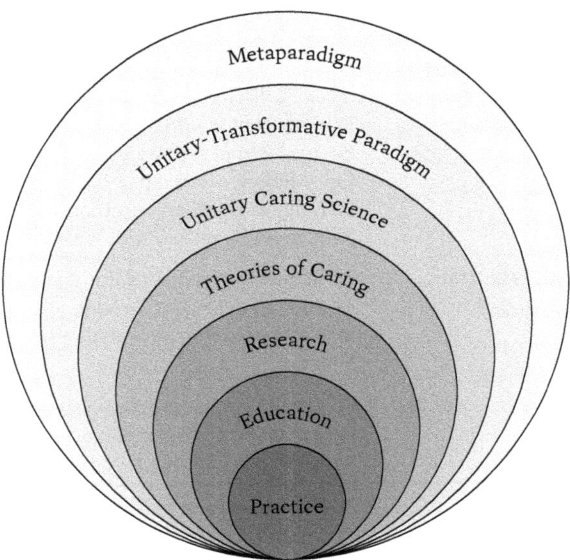


**FIGURE 2.1** Evolution of Praxis within Nursing.

*Note:* Figure 2.1 represents praxis as the interconnectedness of a discipline's worldview, science, theories, research, education, and practice emerging as "a synthesis of thoughtful reflection, caring, and action within theory and research-driven practice (Hines & Gaughan, 2014, p. 26); a synchrony of *knowingdoingbecoming*. Profession (education and practice) is defined within praxis and "consists of persons educated in the [Nursing] discipline according to nationally regulated, defined, and monitored standards" (Parse, 1999, p. 275) for the protection and safety of healthcare for society and its members.

The Unitary-Transformative (UT) Paradigm "acknowledges the irreducible wholeness, connectedness of persons and environment, and the continuous and evolutionary process of [healing] (Kagan et al., 2009, p. 69). Smith and Parker (2020, p. 12) state,

> From the worldview of the unitary-transformative paradigm humans are patterned, self-organizing fields within larger patterned, self-organizing fields. Change is

> characterized by fluctuating rhythms of organization-disorganization toward more complex organization. [Healing] is a reflection of this continuous change.

Therefore, the UT Paradigm presents a worldview where the concepts of reality, change, and the phenomena central to Nursing are uniquely redefined in contrast to our traditional understanding of person, environment, health, and Nurse. Table 2.1 shows this comparison using selected examples.

**TABLE 2.1** Phenomena Central to Nursing—A Comparison

| PHENOMENA | TRADITIONAL PARADIGM | UNITARY-TRANSFORMATIVE PARADIGM |
|---|---|---|
| Person | The sum of parts based on bodily systems | A person is understood as an energyspirit (Phillips, 2015), which is "an irreducible, indivisible, pandimensional energy field identified by pattern and manifesting characteristics that are specific to the whole and which cannot be predicted from knowledge of the parts" (Rogers, 1992, p. 29). |
| Environment | Natural, human/social, physical | Environment is understood as "an irreducible, pandimensional energy field identified by pattern and is integral with the human field" (Rogers, 1992, p. 29). The person-environment field includes everything external to and interacting with person (energyspirit) in a continuous mutual process. |
| Health | Absence of disease; static, understood as existing on a continuum. | Wellbecoming replaces the static concepts of health and wellbeing; a process through which one knowingly participates in changing patterns and manifestations of wholeness and healing. |
| Nurse | Authority figure; illness- and task-focused | Co-creator of healing and peace through unitary caring science; helps person to find meaning in the living experience and well-becoming; soul whisperer, healer. |

Note: *A comparison of phenomena central to Nursing defined within the traditional paradigm and the UT Paradigm with phenomena as defined within the HHE Framework.*

The essence of the phenomena central to Nursing is further illuminated in the UT Paradigm. As person and environment are irreducible and indivisible energy, their pattern and alternating rhythm are in continuous mutual process within a nonlinear domain without spatial or temporal attributes (Rogers, 1992). This is pandimensionality. Within this mutual process, person can knowingly participate in the person-environment field influencing alternating rhythms and the manifestations of pattern. Intention is *choosing* to knowingly participate in the person-environment field.

## Unitary Caring Science and Caring Theories of Nursing

Unitary Caring Science emerges from the UT Paradigm and is congruent with Rogers's Science of Unitary Human Beings (Watson Caring Science Institute, 2021b). Watson tells us that

> Unitary Caring Science is a higher order of thinking beyond Caring Science ... [and] invites an expanded and evolving world view of Unitary or ALL (Watson Caring Science

> Institute, 2021b, para 1, ln 6–7). [Furthermore,] Unitary Caring Science and transpersonal dimensions of the theory of human caring embrace healing arts and humanities, energetic healing practices as moral, timeless philosophically, value-guided praxis. (Watson Caring Institute, 2021b, para 3, ln 4–5).

Theories of Nursing address Nursing's phenomena of interest and guide practice, education, and research—praxis. While theories within the UT Paradigm are philosophically congruent, individual Nursing theorists uniquely define the phenomena of Nursing.

There is a vital link between the UT Paradigm, unitary caring science, caring theories of Nursing, and healing. Therefore, the HHE Framework can be used within any caring theory clustered within the UT Paradigm. While it is beyond the scope of this chapter to describe the many caring theories of Nursing, exemplars of caring theories of Nursing within unitary caring science are presented in Table 2.2.

**TABLE 2.2 Selected Caring Theories of Nursing Congruent within the Unitary-Transformative Paradigm**

| CARING THEORIES OF NURSING—EXEMPLARS | |
|---|---|
| **Theorist** | **Theory Title** |
| Barrett | Theory of Power as Knowing Participation in Change |
| Boykin & Schoenhofer | Theory of Nursing as Caring |
| Dossey | Theory of Integral Nursing |
| Eriksson | Theory of Caritative Caring |
| Falk-Rafael | Critical Caring Theory |
| Newman | Theory of Health as Expanding Consciousness |
| Nightingale | Conceptualizations of Nursing |
| Parse | Humanbecoming Paradigm |
| Ray | Theory of Bureaucratic Caring |
| Reed | Theory of Self-Transcendence |
| Rogers | Science of Unitary Human Beings |
| Smith | Theory of Unitary Caring |
| Swanson | Theory of Caring |
| Watson | Theory of Unitary Caring Science and Theory of Human Caring |

Note: *Exemplars of caring theories of Nursing grounded in the Unitary-Transformative Paradigm (Smith, 2020a).*

## Summary

This chapter presented the development and purpose of the Holistic Healing Environment (HHE) Framework. The evolution of knowledge and praxis within Nursing as a discipline; metaparadigm and phenomena central to Nursing; worldview or paradigm; and selected caring theories of Nursing provide the foundation for understanding the HHE Framework. The purpose of the framework is to guide the Nurse in concert with caring theories of Nursing in co-creating a holistic healing environment within and through caring.

## Key Takeaways from This Chapter

This chapter

- presented the underpinnings of the Holistic Healing Environment (HHE) Framework.
- The HHE Framework is grounded in the Unitary-Transformative Paradigm and Unitary Caring Science and is integral with caring theories of Nursing clustered within the Unitary-Transformative Paradigm.
- Nurses guiding their praxis with caring theories of Nursing can integrate the HHE Framework to co-create a holistic healing environment where healing emerges within and through caring.

## End-of-Chapter Questions, Applications, and Group Activities

**Directions:** Use what you have learned in this chapter to reflect upon and respond to the questions and prompts below.

### Questions

1. Why is it important for Nursing to have a unique paradigm from other disciplines?
2. What are the phenomena central to Nursing?
3. How is the phenomenon of wellbecoming different from the concepts of health and wellbeing?

### Applications

1. Choose a caring theory of Nursing from Table 2.1. Read through the theory description on the Nursology website.

**Nursology: Caring Theories to Choose From**

**WEB LINK:** https://nursology.net/

Identify areas or components of the theory that resonate with how you see the world and/or your practice and where you believe healing may emerge through caring.

2. Review Orem's Self-Care Deficit Nursing Theory. Is it congruent with the UT Paradigm? Why or why not?

## Group Activities

1. Each group member selects a health care discipline other than Nursing (medicine, respiratory therapy, social work, etc.). Then the group compares and contrasts the phenomena of interest across disciplines including Nursing.

3

# The Holistic Healing Environment Framework

*Holistic Healing Environment—noun: Dance of alternating rhythms with intentional knowing participation to co-create an environment through which holistic healing emerges for Nurse and person(s).*

## Introduction

This chapter presents the Holistic Healing Environment (HHE) Framework—its focus, purpose, and its integration into praxis. The framework is grounded in the Unitary-Transformative (UT) Paradigm and is central to Nursing as a discipline, science, art, and profession as described in Chapters 1 and 2. Before getting started, however, we invite you to write a reflection on the following question:

What do you already know or think about curing? Healing?

Just a gentle reminder—there are no incorrect answers! After you finish, set your writing aside and move on to the rest of the chapter.

### Objectives

After completing this chapter, readers will:

- Differentiate between curing and healing.
- Describe the HHE Framework.
- Within the HHE Framework, describe the call for Nursing.

### Key Terms and Concepts

**Directions:** Before continuing reading, take time to become familiar with key concepts integral to the HHE Framework included in this chapter.

- **Healing**—Personal experience of transcending suffering; a pandimensional, nonlinear emergent mutual process of the integrality of one's *heartmindbodysoul* and environment.

- **Wellbecoming**—A process through which one knowingly participates in changing patterns and manifestations of wholeness.
- **Knowing participation**—The intentional mutual patterning within person and environment, which are unitary and inseparable.
- **Patterns of knowing**—Are manifested as repeating/enduring waves of *knowingdoingbecoming* that are always integral, evolving, and emerging.
- ***Knowingdoingbecoming***—Manifests the wholeness and alternating rhythms of healing *heartmindbodysoul.*
- **Intention**—The choice to knowingly participate in the person-environment field.
- **Authentic presence**—Awareness of and coming to know self in synchrony and harmony within alternating rhythms guided by Mayeroff's ingredients of caring and Roach's caring attributes to choose *who I bring to practice in this moment.*
- **Integral presence**—"A perceiving-experiencing of the integrality of [persons] and the environment" (Phillips, 2015, p. 46) emerging from authentic presence, as the Nurse experiences the wholeness of self and other and the interconnectedness of self with other.
- **Compassionate unity**—Emerges within integral presence and is the alternating rhythms of perceiving-experiencing *I feel you, you feel me, and I feel you feeling me* (Hübl, 2021, p. 2); the interwoven energy field of Nurse and other, simultaneously the healer and healee—both healing and both being healed. Within compassionate unity, Nurse is soul whisperer and healer.
- **Soul whisperer**—Nurse interconnects with person soul-to-soul through "pandimensional thoughts such as soothing, tender, quieting, and loving, giving illumination and radiance" (Phillips, 2015, p. 46) to transcend suffering.

## The Soul of the Holistic Healing Environment (HHE) Framework

Healing is influenced by environment, which includes everything external to and interacting with person (energyspirit). Within the Holistic Healing Environment (HHE) Framework, the focus of Nursing is healing. Therefore, *the call for Nursing* is to co-create an environment of holistic healing for the Nurse and other to transcend suffering. The purpose of the framework is to guide the Nurse in concert within caring theories of Nursing in co-creating a holistic healing environment where healing emerges within and through caring. What then is a holistic healing environment? A holistic healing environment, within the HHE Framework, is the dance of alternating rhythms with intentional knowing participation to co-create an environment through which holistic healing emerges for Nurse and person(s).

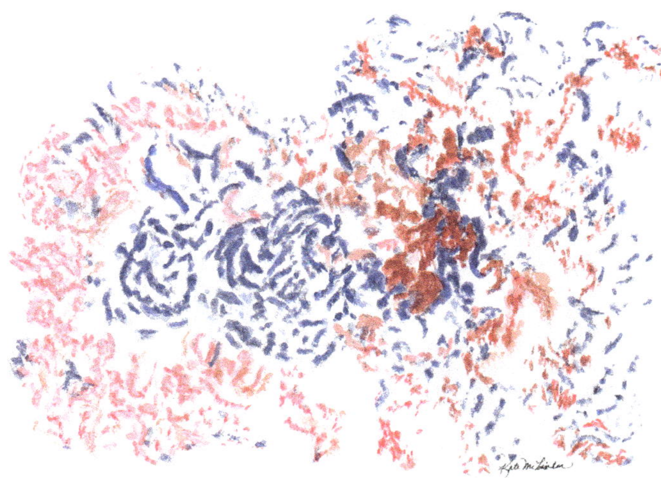

**FIGURE 3.1** Holistic Healing Environment Framework. Kathleen McLinden, "Holistic Healing Environment Framework." Copyright © by Shirley C. Gordon and Nancey E.M. France. Reprinted with permission.

The HHE Framework does not stand by itself but is philosophically congruent with caring theories of Nursing in the Unitary-Transformative Paradigm. The following section describes the soul (emotional/intellectual energy) of the framework: the unique focus of Nursing, the call for Nursing, mutual process and knowing participation, *knowingdoingbecoming* as mutual patterning, and integration into praxis.

## The Unique Focus of Nursing: Healing

Within the HHE Framework, the unique focus of Nursing is healing emerging through and within caring. Wellbecoming is a manifestation of healing, and neither are synonymous with curing. Curing is understood as "the elimination of the signs and symptoms of disease, which may or may not even correspond to the end of the patient's disease or distress" (Quinn, 2022, p. 101). Curing may occur without healing and healing may occur without curing.

"Healing comes from the etymological root, *haele* or *haelen*, the Anglo-Saxon word meaning whole or having integrity" (Smith et al., 2013, p. 174). Within the HHE Framework, healing is defined as a personal experience of transcending suffering, a nonlinear emergent mutual process of the integrality of one's *heartmindbodysoul* and environment where the person as energyspirit and environment simultaneously experience healing—both the Nurse and the other are healed. "In the end, healing may be, like pain, what the patient says it is" (Quinn, 2017, p. 269).

Wellbecoming is a process through which one knowingly participates in changing patterns and manifestations of wholeness and healing. It replaces the concept of health and wellbeing and is always emerging and evolving. Therefore, wellbecoming is not understood as existing on a continuum.

The Nurse is integral to healing through co-creating a holistic healing environment. A holistic healing environment is not a physical place, space, or architecture. As described in Chapter 2, environment includes everything external to and interacting with person (energyspirit), where healing emerges from the integrality of *knowingdoingbecoming* as the mutual patterning within person and environment.

## The Call for Nursing

Within the HHE Framework, the call for Nursing is to co-create a holistic healing environment through which healing emerges for Nurse and person(s). The call for Nursing is not when the Nurse responds to the call light or fulfills a task such as getting the patient a drink or turning the patient. The call is how the Nurse responds to or fulfills Nursing care *when integrally present and within compassionate unity.* Within integral presence and compassionate unity, Nurse as soul whisperer and healer comes to know the call for Nursing to co-create a holistic healing environment.

Soul whisperer and healer are a sacred manifestation of caring. Within compassionate unity, the Nurse as soul whisperer and healer experiences/perceives a deeper pandimensional mutual knowing of another's soul to transcend suffering. For example, when we touch another's body, we are simultaneously touching the mind, the heart, and the soul with "pandimensional thoughts such as soothing, tender, quieting and loving" (Phillips, 2015, p. 28). The call for Nursing in *any* Nursing Situation is experienced only through compassionate unity, which emerges through mutual process, knowing participation, and *knowingdoingbecoming.*

## Mutual Process and Knowing Participation

A basic premise of the framework is that we are in continuous mutual process with each other either knowingly or unknowingly. Unknowing participation is how we typically go through our day. We are focused on self, the tasks we need to accomplish, and our basic physical needs (when to eat, sleep, etc.), without much thought on how we influence or impact another person's day, feelings, or mood.

We may not realize, for example, if our communication is more curt than usual because we had a rough morning carrying this with us to our day and to those with whom we come in contact. How many times have we said, "Well, that person got up on the wrong side of the bed this morning"? Have you ever been with a small group of people who were all having a good time and someone joined the group who was in a bad mood? What happened to the group's energy field? Did it shift from positive to negative? Now imagine as Nurse you are experiencing a difficult day. How might the quality of care your patients receive be impacted?

The human energy field and environmental energy field are distinct but not separate. Each field is manifested by a pattern that represents "the distinguishing characteristic of an energy field perceived as a single wave" (Rogers, 1992, p. 29). As human energy fields, our thoughts, emotions, words, and nonverbal actions are in continuous mutual process with our environment—person-to-person, Nurse-to-patient, and so on. While we cannot prevent this interaction, persons can choose to *knowingly* participate within our environment and intentionally co-create a holistic healing environment. Knowing participation is intentional. Intention is the *choice* to knowingly participate within the person-environment field. Knowing participation is mutual patterning within person and environment, which are unitary and inseparable (Butcher & Malinski, 2020). Through knowing participation and mutual patterning, change occurs simultaneously for person and environment (Butcher & Malinski, 2020).

## *Knowingdoingbecoming* as Mutual Patterning

*Knowingdoingbecoming* as mutual patterning manifests the wholeness and alternating rhythms of healing and is integral to caring for self, authentic presence, integral presence and compassionate unity. Mayeroff's ingredients of caring, Roach's attributes of caring, and patterns of knowing are foundational to *knowingdoingbecoming*. The following paragraphs describe each one separately but *knowingdoingbecoming* is complex and pandimensional. Students are encouraged to read the original works of Mayeroff, Roach, and the patterns of knowing.

## Ingredients of Caring

Mayeroff (1971) was a sociologist who published a classic work on caring. The purpose of his work was to explore/define the *meaning* of caring in one's own life as well as by serving others through caring. Mayeroff (1971) carefully describes a mutual process in helping another to grow and experience transformation in wholeness through identified caring ingredients: knowing, alternating rhythms, patience, honesty, trust, humility, hope, and courage. Within the HHE Framework, this mutual process is fundamental to healing. *Nurse as soul whisperer and healer* starts with the Nurse holistically caring-for-self as energyspirit following **Mayeroff's (1971) ingredients of caring**—knowing, alternating rhythms, patience, honesty, trust, humility, hope, and courage. This means having the courage, patience, and humility to be honest in coming to know self in alternating rhythms and having trust and hope during this daily journey. Table 3.1 presents definitions of the ingredients of caring.

**TABLE 3.1** Mayeroff's Ingredients of Caring

| INGREDIENT | DEFINITION |
|---|---|
| Knowing | Simultaneously experienced as explicit, implicit, direct, and indirect. Explicit knowing is being able "to tell what we know, ... put into words" (Mayeroff, 1971, p. 20). Implicit knowing is being unable to clearly articulate what we know. Direct knowing is experiencing, encountering someone or something in individuality and not as a stereotype. Indirect knowing is having information without directly experiencing. Knowing is simultaneous and pandimensional—we cannot reduce it as this then restricts the meaning of knowing and knowledge. |
| Alternating rhythms | The rhythm and pattern of moving back and forth, narrow and wider; as part and as whole; reflective and reflexive. |
| Patience | Mutual participation with the other, giving time, space, and respect to self and other. |
| Honesty | "Actively confronting and being open to oneself" (Mayeroff, 1971, p. 25); genuineness; "no significant gap between how I act and what I really feel, between what I say and what I feel" (p. 26). |
| Trust | In myself—"confidence in my judgments and my ability to learn from mistakes" (Mayeroff, 1971, p. 29). "Trusting the other is to let go; includes an element of risk ... a leap into the unknown" (p. 27). Trust takes courage. |
| Humility | "Overcoming pretentiousness ... to present myself as I am," "a truer appreciation of my limitations" (Mayeroff, 1971, p. 31). |
| Hope | "An expression of a present alive with possibilities. ... Not wishful thinking and unfounded expectations ... not a passive waiting for something to happen from outside" (Mayeroff, 1971, pp. 30, 31). |
| Courage | "Going into the unknown" (Mayeroff, 1971, p. 34). |

Note: *This is a brief presentation to capture the essence of Mayeroff's ingredients of caring. Readers are strongly encouraged to read his original work.*

## Attributes of Caring

While Mayeroff defined the meaning of caring within a sociological perspective, Roach explicated the meaning of caring in Nursing practice. As a Nurse, she asserted that "caring is the human mode of being" (Roach, 2002, p. 38) and asked what is the Nurse doing when he/she is caring? Roach's attributes of caring (compassion, competence, confidence, conscience, commitment, and comportment), commonly known as the 6 Cs, suggest categories of caring behaviors within which caring in Nursing can be understood. "Compassionate and competent acts, in relationships, qualified by confidence, through informed sensitive conscience, and through commitment and fidelity" (2002, p. 66) are lived moment-to-moment as the Nurse co-creates a holistic healing environment. Table 3.2 presents Roach's attributes of caring.

**TABLE 3.2** Roach's Attributes of Caring

| ATTRIBUTE | DEFINITION |
|---|---|
| Compassion | "... a way of living born out of an awareness of one's relationship to all living creatures" (Roach, 2002, p. 50). |
| Competence | "The state of having the knowledge, judgment, skills, energy, experience and motivation required to respond adequately to the demands of one's professional responsibilities" (Roach, 2002, p. 54). |
| Confidence | "... the quality that fosters trusting relationships" (Roach, 2002, p. 56). |
| Conscience | "... the morally sensitive self attuned to values, is integral to personhood; reflects the sacredness of the person, points to the sacred core of the personality and to the centre of personal integrity" (Roach, 2002, p. 58). |
| Commitment | "... a complex affective response characterized by a convergence between one's desires and one's obligations, and by a deliberate choice to act in accordance with them" (Roach, 2002, p. 62). |
| Comportment | "Are dress and language of caregivers consistent with the belief that the patient-client is of incalculable worth, and that the caregiver him-/herself is a person of intrinsic worth and dignity?" (Roach, 2002, p. 65). |

Note: *This is a brief presentation to capture the essence of Roach's attributes of caring. Readers are strongly encouraged to read her original work.*

## Patterns of Knowing

Patterns of knowing form the structure of the discipline, inform Nursing praxis, and support coming to know self and other. Within the HHE Framework, in Nursing, patterns of knowing are manifested as repeating/enduring waves of *knowingdoingbecoming* that are always integral, evolving, and emerging.

While Mayeroff identified knowing as an ingredient of caring, Carper was the first scholar to identify patterns of knowing in Nursing based on a review of Nursing curricula. The patterns of knowing identified in her writings and scholarly works were empirical, aesthetic, ethical, and personal (Carper, 1978). Over time, additional patterns of knowing have continued to emerge: emancipatory (Chinn & Kramer, 2018); spiritual (Willis & Leone-Sheehan, 2019), sociopolitical (White, 1995), narrative (Sandelowski, 1991), intuition (McCraty, Atkinson, & Bradley, 2004;) technological (Lim-Saco, Kilat, & Locsin, 2018); and unknowing (Munhall, 1993). Table 3.3 presents an exemplar of patterns of knowing.

**TABLE 3.3** Exemplars of the Patterns of Knowing

| PATTERN | DEFINITION |
|---|---|
| Empirical (Carper, 1978) | "... knowledge that is systematically organized into general laws and theories for the purpose of describing, explaining and predicting phenomena ..." (p. 14). |
| Personal (Carper 1978) | "... concerned with the knowing, encountering and actualizing of the concrete individual self" (p. 18). |
| Aesthetic (Rogers, 1988) | Aesthetics, a pattern of knowing, is concerned with the art of Nursing. The art of Nursing is "the imaginative and creative use of knowledge" (p. 100). |
| Ethical (Carper, 1978) | "The fundamental patterns of knowing identified here as the ethical component of Nursing is focused on matters of obligation or what ought to be done" (p. 20). |
| Spiritual (Willis & Leone-Sheehan, 2019) | The "human beings' perceiving and appreciating of nonmaterial spiritual qualities and experiences that provide meaning and purpose, awareness of a greater reality, and uplifting of the human spirit" (p. 62). |
| Emancipatory (Chinn & Kramer, 2018) | "... focuses on developing an awareness of social problems and taking action to create social change" (p. 2). |
| Sociopolitical (White, 1995) | Addresses the "wherein"—"lifts the gaze of the Nurse from the introspective Nurse-patient relationship and situates it within the broader context in which Nursing and healthcare take place" (p. 83). Sociopolitical knowing involves the "sociopolitical context of the persons (Nurse and patient) and the sociopolitical context of Nursing as a practice profession, including both society's understanding of Nursing and Nursing's understanding of society and its politics" (p. 84). |
| Narrative (Sandelowski, 1994) | "The knowledge transmitted in the stories that human beings have told each other since the beginning" (p. 23). |
| Intuition (McCraty, Atkinson, & Bradley, 2004) | "... a process by which information normally outside the range of conscious awareness is perceived by the psychophysiological systems" (p. 133). |
| Technological (Lim-Saco, Kilat, & Locsin, 2018) | "... focused on providing authentic and humane caring. Guided by technology, ... is the process that leads the Nurse in sensing relevant data and pattern information about the Nursed in interaction as persons and not as objects of care" (p. 7). |
| Unknowing | choosing to be open in *heartmindbodysoul* to come-to-know other in the moment. |

Note: *Exemplars of patterns of knowing currently identified in the Nursing literature.*

While each ingredient of caring, each attribute of caring, and each pattern of knowing is necessary, they are not sufficient when used individually. Within alternating rhythms, the ingredients of caring, attributes of caring, and patterns of knowing in their entirety are understood to be necessary to guide *Nursing practice.* Within the HHE Framework, Myeroff's ingredients of caring, Roach's attributes of caring, and patterns of knowing are understood as a unified whole, integral to *knowingdoingbecoming* and necessary for guiding *Nursing praxis.*

As described earlier, *knowingdoingbecoming* as mutual patterning manifests the wholeness and alternating rhythms of healing within Mayeroff's ingredients of caring, Roach's attributes of caring, and patterns of knowing. This mutual patterning is integral to caring for self, authentic presence, integral presence, and compassionate unity.

**Thoughtful Reflection**

Are compassion and compassionate unity the same?

Within the HHE Framework, compassion and compassionate unity are not the same. Compassion is a commonly used concept within Nursing. For example, compassion is generally defined as "the feeling or emotion, when a person is moved by the suffering or distress of another, and by the desire to relieve it" (Simpson, Weiner, & Oxford University Press, 1988, 2a.) Within the six caring attributes, Roach always listed compassion first. She described compassion as a way of living that "engenders a response of participation in the experience of another ... and a quality of presence that allows one to share with and make room for the other" (2002, p. 50).

Compassion, within the HHE Framework, is experienced when the Nurse is authentically present. Authentic Presence is the awareness of and coming to know self in synchrony and harmony within alternating rhythms guided by Mayeroff's ingredients of caring and Roach's caring attributes to choose *who I bring to practice in this moment*.

Integral presence emerges from authentic presence. It is a perceiving-experiencing of the integrality of the person-environment field (Phillips, 2015), as the Nurse experiences the wholeness of self and other and the interconnectedness of self with other.

Compassionate unity emerges within integral presence. It is the alternating rhythms of perceiving-experiencing *I feel you, you feel me, and I feel you feeling me* (Hübl, 2021, p. 2)—the interwoven energy field of Nurse and other, simultaneously the healer and healee, both healing and both being healed. It is within compassionate unity, Nurse is soul whisperer and healer.

## Integration in Nursing Praxis

In this section we will use a Nursing Situation to reveal the integration of the HHE Framework in Nursing praxis. This Nursing Situation unfolds in a middle school setting in which the Nurse focuses on the care of a student with diabetes. It begins with the Nurse practicing within the traditional paradigm and then comes to know how she was not authentically present or knowingly participating.

# Nursing Situation: Forever Changed

*As a Nurse working in the school health setting, I provide care to children and adolescents who live with chronic health conditions. Type 1 diabetes is a chronic health condition that requires daily care in the school health clinic requiring close monitoring and management.*

*I was asked to float to a middle school to cover for a Nurse for approximately eight weeks. One of the seventh-grade students that I received a report on was a young man named Sean living with Type 1 diabetes since he was five years old. I was given a report that he would not follow directives, blood glucose levels were elevated, he would not rotate his injections sites, and he would come to the clinic frequently to get out of going to class. My very first day working in the clinic, Sean was sent home due to an elevated blood glucose level.*

*My goal was to promote self-care of his diabetes. I would need to reinforce education regarding hyperglycemia and hypoglycemia because he lived with high blood glucose levels and frequently required correction doses. I took the time and effort to explain the importance of counting and reporting carbohydrates, not sneaking extra snacks at lunch, keeping water on himself during the school day, and taking insulin doses as directed.*

*I even brought in every extra water bottle I had in my house and stored them in the clinic. When he came into the clinic prior to breakfast, I would fill it up and give it to him. Throughout the day I encouraged him to maintain proper hydration. I would have the cafeteria menus with carbohydrate counts on the refrigerator. I expected him to look at the menu every morning, decide on his meals, and be directly involved with counting the carbs and correction dose if needed. He was expected to calculate his insulin dose on his calculator—not just the Nurse counting it all together and providing him the number.*

*But there was a lot of push back and defiant behavior—a manifestation of Sean's* ***unknowing participation****. I have had many experiences in different age groups, but this one situation was one that even though I thought I was* ***authentically present,*** *I could not engage with this young man as I, too, was unknowingly participating. Upon reflection, I realized that I had been so focused on teaching him self-care strategies that I was not focused on coming to know Sean in his wholeness. I had not set my intention on who I chose to bring to practice in the moment. Therefore, I realized I was not* ***authentically*** *or* ***integrally present****.*

*From that day on, in integral presence, I experienced wholeness of myself and him and the interconnectedness of myself with him. I then saw a pattern—Sean was angry with his diagnosis and viewed diabetes as a threat to his wellbecoming. Instead of starting our meeting in the clinic focused on his diabetes, I was aware of our alternating rhythms and open to him as person as energyspirit—asking him how his day was going so far, or how his night was. As we experienced alternating rhythms of perceiving-experiencing, we were in compassionate unity, and he began to open up with me. I learned he was the oldest child. He told me his mother had to take care of his two young twin brothers at home as his father left a year ago. So Sean was mainly self-managing his chronic health condition on his own. He was responsible to take his long-acting insulin at home and cover accordingly for insulin correction.*

*He started talking to me about other things than his diagnosis—what classes he liked and did not like and the crush he had on a girl in one of his classes. He told me he felt sad a lot of the time and worried about his mom and brothers. Conversation on weekend plans or what he wanted to do to celebrate his birthday became a daily part of our routine.*

*Through* ***compassionate unity,*** *there was mutual patterning, and he was* ***knowingly participating*** *in caring for self. I noticed a positive change in Sean from that first week in the clinic. The first time he came in with a normal blood glucose level in the morning and did not require an insulin adjustment was a defining moment for both of us. We celebrated with a glass of unsweetened iced tea!*

*During my last week at this middle school, Sean brought a poem he had written for me. With a big smile, he told me, "Even though you're my Nurse, I consider us friends, too."*

*As Sean had experienced mutual patterning change, I, too, was forever changed as a Nurse.*

**Thoughtful Reflection**

How does the Nurse become authentically present and emerge from authentic presence to integral presence and from integral presence to compassionate unity?

In Chapter 1, "Nurse as Soul Whisperer and Healer," how Nurse becomes authentically present with intention and emerges from authentic presence to integral presence was described. As Nurse focuses on inner coherence, he/she then experiences the wholeness of self. The Nurse holistically cares for self as energyspirit following Mayeroff's ingredients of caring—knowing, alternating rhythms, patience, honesty, trust, humility, hope, and courage. This means having the courage, patience, and humility to be honest in coming to know self in alternating rhythms and having trust and hope during this daily journey. Coming to know is having awareness of who *you choose to bring to practice in that moment.* Holding that awareness within alternating rhythms and now being guided with Roach's 6 Cs is authentic presence.

Person unknowingly participates in his/her healing. Nurse as soul whisperer and healer is knowingly participating, becoming authentically present, then integrally present. Through authentic presence, the Nurse knowingly becomes open to experiencing the interconnectedness of self with other—a perceiving-experiencing of the integrality of the person-environment field (Phillips, 2015) known as integral presence through which compassionate unity emerges. When the Nurse is integrally present, he/she and other are simultaneously healer and healee through their wholeness and openness—there is no fragmentation, and there is no compassion fatigue as may be experienced in authentic presence. As the Nurse's energy is integral with person's energy, within compassionate unity the Nurse and other are knowingly participating and experience *I feel you, you feel me, and I feel you feeling me* (Hübl, 2021, p. 2) simultaneously. It is through knowing participation and mutual patterning that change occurs simultaneously and healing emerges (Butcher & Malinski, 2020). Within compassionate unity, as Nurse and other are both healing and being healed, they are co-creating a holistic healing environment. We invite you to reflect on the artist's rendition of the HHE Framework represented in Figure 3.2.

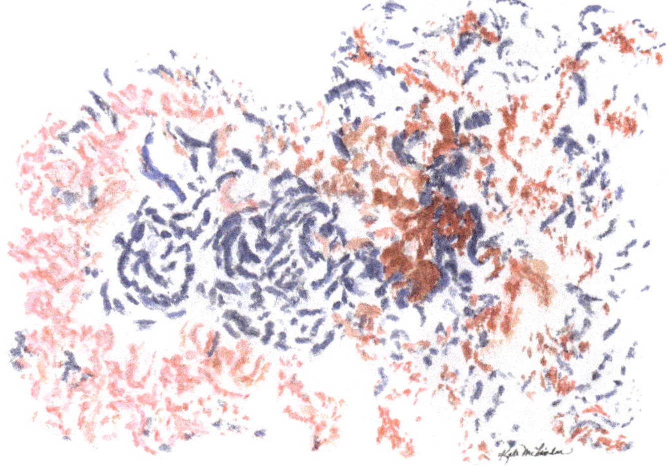

FIGURE 3.2 Artist's Rendition of the Holistic Healing Framework Framework. Kathleen McLinden, "Holistic Healing Environment Framework." Copyright © by Shirley C. Gordon and Nancey E.M. France. Reprinted with permission.

On the left, you will see swirls of energy—the pink represents the Nurse as energyspirit within gentle authentic and integral presence; the blue represents the energyspirit of the other person seeking calm and healing. Nurse and person are in continuous mutual process—the Nurse knowingly participating, and person unknowingly participating. Within authentic presence, the Nurse has awareness of and comes to know self in synchrony and harmony within alternating rhythms guided by Mayeroff's ingredients of caring and Roach's caring attributes to choose *who I bring to practice in this moment.* Following the patterns and alternating rhythms toward the center, you experience the Nurse as energyspirit transitioning from authentic presence to integral presence with more pink and increasing brilliance of the person/patient as energyspirit (blue). Beautiful shades transitioning from pink to red reveal the mutual process and alternating rhythms that portray "a perceiving-experiencing of the integrality of [persons] and the environment" (Phillips, 2015, p. 46) as the Nurse experiences the wholeness of self and other and the interconnectedness of self with other. Within this integral presence emerges compassionate unity captured in the deepening richness of red—the alternating rhythms of perceiving-experiencing *I feel you, you feel me, and I feel you feeling me* (Hübl, 2021, p. 2)—the interwoven energy field of Nurse and other simultaneously the healer and healee, both healing and both being healed. The power of compassionate unity is portrayed emerging with radiance and transcending suffering.

## Summary

This chapter presented the essence of the Holistic Healing Environment (HHE) Framework and guides Nurse and other in co-creating healing. The framework is grounded in the Unitary-Transformative (UT) Paradigm and is central to Nursing as a discipline, science, art, and profession. The artist's rendition in Figure 3.1 illuminates the power of compassionate unity emerging with radiance and transcending suffering.

## Key Takeaways from This Chapter

Below is a list of key information and ideas to take away from your reading.

- The essence of the HHE Framework is to describe how Nurse and other co-create healing.
- The HHE Framework does not stand by itself but is philosophically congruent with caring theories of Nursing in the Unitary-Transformative Paradigm.
- Within the HHE Framework, the focus of Nursing is healing.
- The call for Nursing is to co-create an HHE for the Nurse and person to transcend suffering through and within healing.
- Curing, healing and wellbecoming are not synonymous.
- Wellbecoming is a manifestation of healing.
- The Nurse holds the awareness of coming to know self in synchrony and harmony within alternating rhythms guided by Mayeroff's ingredients of caring and Roach's caring attributes to become authentically present and choose *who I bring to practice in this moment.*
- Patterns of knowing are manifested as repeating/enduring waves of *knowingdoingbecoming* that are always integral, evolving, and emerging.

- The Nurse emerges from authentic presence to integral presence to experience compassionate unity with the other.
- The Nurse as soul whisperer and healer is a sacred manifestation of caring.

# End-of-Chapter Questions, Applications, and Group Activities

**Directions:** Use what you have learned in this chapter to reflect upon and respond to the questions and prompts below.

## Questions and Reflections

- In your own words, explain the difference between curing, healing, and wellbecoming. Give an example of each.
- Describe your understanding of knowing participation.
- Reflect on a personal experience of unknowingly participating. How could you change that to knowingly participating?
- Ask yourself, who do I choose to bring to practice in this moment? Journal your reflection.

## Applications

- Write a Nursing Situation from your practice. Describe how you would apply the HHE Framework to this Nursing Situation.
- Take a moment to look again at the artist's painting of the Framework. What do you see now? How has your perception changed?
- Based on the Nursing Situation described in this chapter, create the poem you think Sean would have written for the Nurse.

## Group Activities

- In Chapter 1, you were presented with a Nursing Situation. Let's revisit it—read it again and apply the HHE Framework.
  - Ask yourself "How did the Nurse come to know the call for Nursing to co-create a holistic healing environment?"

# UNIT II

# Co-Creating a Holistic Healing Environment

## *Nurses' Living Experiences*

## Introduction

In this unit, we provide an opportunity to reflect upon selected Nurses' living experiences within which the Holistic Healing Environment (HHE) Framework is manifested. Through discovering the patterns of knowing and ingredients of caring, we come to understand the emergence of *knowingdoingbecoming* and compassionate unity.

The HHE Framework can be used with any caring theory of Nursing within the Unitary-Transformative (UT) Paradigm. In this unit, we will challenge you to engage in the reflective reflexive process of moving between and within philosophy and theory (abstract ideas and concepts) and practice exemplar (specific, concrete phenomena) and returning to philosophy and theory through the HHE Framework. See Figure II.1 for a visual representation of the reflective reflexive process.

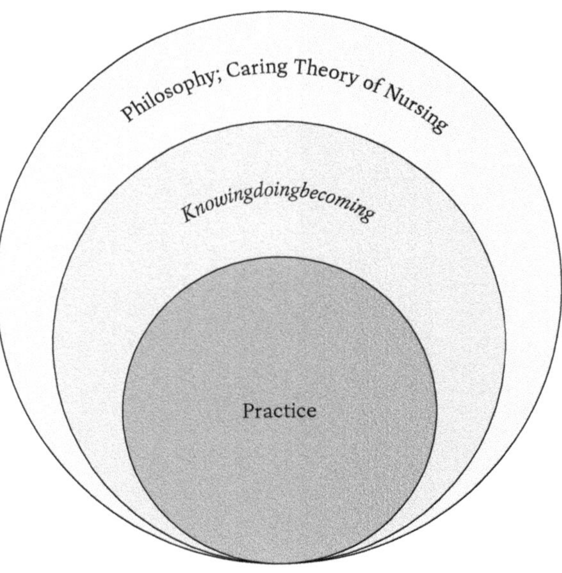


**FIGURE II.1** Reflective Reflexive Process.
Note: *Knowingdoingbecoming is central to the reflective reflexive process within the HHE Framework.*

Each chapter in this unit is based on conversational interviews with Nurses who practice from a holistic foundation in a variety of settings. We invited each Nurse to share the following with us:

1. Describe an exemplar from practice, a Nursing Situation, in which you co-created an environment that supported healing.

a. How did you experience healing?
b. How did the patient/client experience healing?

2. What is an essential element for co-creating a healing environment in your practice?
3. What do you think is important for Nurses to know as they begin to co-create a healing environment in their practice?

Watson invites us to conceptualize Nurse's work as sacred (Watson, Malking & Alvarez, 2014). The Nursing Situations in this unit represent this sacred work through Nurses' living experiences of co-creating a holistic healing environment in practice. As each Nurse shares a story about a past event, he/she relives the event and all the phenomena around and within that event. Therefore, an event experienced in the past continues being experienced in the present—as living. As the Nurses shared their stories, they were reliving their experiences. Their shared living experiences live on through you!

4

# "I Trust You"

## Introduction

In this chapter, we introduce you to Mary Enzman Hines, PhD, APRN, CNS, CPNP-PC, APHN-BC, SGAHN, known as Dr. Mary to everyone in her care. Among her vast educational preparation, Dr. Mary is a board-certified pediatric Nurse practitioner, advanced holistic Nurse, Reiki master, and Nurse scholar/researcher and has 48 years of clinical practice experience. She is a Founding Scholar Global Academy of Holistic Nursing and co-owner of Integrative Pediatric Health Care, LLC. *"I was different than most people and I always wanted to be a Nurse since I was five. I said to my mother, when I was five, I was going to be a Nurse. She said, Yeah, well, nobody's been a Nurse in our family so forget that and you better find something else.' I mean I've been a holistic Nurse, since I was five ... because I was called"* (Hines, personal communication, December 10, 2021).

Early on in practice, however, Dr. Mary realized that *"most of what the medical and Nursing profession does is alienate those poor children because we want them all to fit into a little box and a diagnosis. And what they want to be as children is normal; they want to be regarded for who they are. So that's really resonated with me—this whole idea of relation-based caring and how you approach care in a healing dynamic"* (Hines, personal communication, December 10, 2021).

> *I experience healing every day with the smiles on those children's faces and the hugs they give me. When they come in, parents will say, "They've been talking about Dr. Mary in the car for miles. Before we got here, 'We're going to see Dr. Mary today.'" So that's what I try to create—an environment where when parents come in as a new patient, they'll notice that too, that I'm talking to the child. The child is my patient, you are their parent—you certainly have a historicity with them, you certainly have a lot of information I need. But I'm going to be talking to your child and I do that from the time they're tiny babies. Those parents just laugh at me. They say, "You pick them up, and you have a whole conversation with them." And that's right, because you can see through their eyes. They don't need to have language. You can see through their eyes what they need and want. And I try to teach parents that if you would just pay more attention to their cues and less to that social media that tells you how to be a parent and really tune into your child, your child will tell you what they need.* (Hines, personal communication, December 10, 2021)

We asked Dr. Mary, from her perspective, what is an essential element for co-creating a holistic healing environment in practice. She was very clear.

> *So, you've got to pay attention to the environment. I learned that from a very young Nurse in the PICU [pediatric intensive care unit] that you could really shift the environment in those rooms by simply the lighting and just calming people. Like I would have Nurses come in, and I would be in charge in the PICU and they'd say, "This is going to be just a horrible night." I'd say, "Okay, let's all kind of come up here to the to the desk. We're going to get into a caring circle here and we're going to talk about this, because this is not how we're going to do this night. These patients are critically ill, and they need you to be present with them. They don't need you to bring in your stuff, okay? So, let's all kind of refocus here." And that's where kind of our ideas of huddles came long before we had the caring huddles. I did that very early in the military. I mean we huddled together—we went through a lot together. So, I think you've got to shift those environments when you're feeling that negativity. And you can feel it with patients sometimes. They'll say something and I'll say, "I'm feeling some tenseness here. Can we talk a little bit about what's happening here?" Because if you let that go on, that's when those confrontational kind of experiences happen. And I explained to every patient, "I'm not here to tell you what to do. I'm here to open the possibilities and the ways that it can be done and you're going to be the decision maker for your child. You always will be, as you're the parent."* (Hines, personal communication, December 10, 2021)

Dr. Mary shared an exemplar from her private practice that described how she pays attention to the environment for two- and three-year-olds making it safe:

> *So, what I do first off, I use books a lot. I bring books in, and we use picture books and I bring in certain things that will distract them. And I sing a lot. I sing to the kids because they know music, so we will oftentimes get into singing. Sometimes they like hugs; they want to sit on my lap, so we'll sit, and we'll hug, and I let them play with my instruments (otoscope, stethoscope). So, I let them play with instruments before I listen, we can listen to their music that they brought in, or I provide something. I let them manipulate things. I make that environment safe, because if you just go in and charge a child that's how they'll respond.* (Hines, personal communication, December 10, 2021)

**Thoughtful Reflections**

Reflect upon Dr. Mary's understanding of the importance of *relation-based caring and "how you approach care in a healing dynamic."* How does this idea resonate within your practice?

## Objectives

After completing this chapter, readers will:

- Within the Nurse's living experience described in this chapter, identify the patterns of knowing and ingredients of caring.

- Within the HHE Framework, describe the Nurse's *knowingdoingbecoming* as soul whisperer and healer in the context of the Nursing Situation described above.
- Demonstrate the reflective reflexive process in applying the HHE Framework within the selected Nursing Situation.

### Key Terms and Concepts

**Directions:** Before continuing, we encourage you to take time to become familiar with key concepts integral to understanding Nurses' living experience in co-creating a holistic healing environment.

- **Grounding**—"The process of connecting to the earth and the earth's energy field to calm the mind and focus one's inner flow of energy as a means to enhance healing endeavors" (Thornton & Mariano, 2022, p. 368); illuminates an awareness of the unity of *heartmindbodysoul.*
- **Centering**—An intentional process of becoming authentically present to self within *heartmindbodysoul.*
- **Caring circle**—Co-creating space through awareness of self within alternating rhythms to strengthen a sense of community from which emerges synchronous authentic presence.
- **Reiki**—Is "spiritually guided life energy" (New York Presbyterian Hospital, 2022, par. 4) connecting us with our environment. As an energy therapy, persons may experience relaxation, peacefulness, calmness, and wellbecoming. Reiki therapy can involve touch or no touch.

## Nursing Situation: "*I Trust You*"

Dr. Mary shared the following Nursing Situation.

> *I'll tell you a little bit about Anna. She was a seven-year-old, who came into my office probably about six months after I started practice and she had come from [the Northeast] with her mother. Her mother had been terribly abused by a violent partner and was very traumatized. I couldn't even get much eye contact with her during the first visit because she was so afraid of what I might ask. So, Anna was coming in with abdominal pain, which is my common chronic complaint of children who've been through trauma. The mother had labeled her as having a lot of anxiety and lack of focus and was wondering if maybe she had ADHD or maybe she was really constipated. She came up with this laundry list of stuff because she said she'd been on the Internet.*
>
> *And I just looked for a moment and I said, You know energetically this room is tense to me. Are you guys feeling that?*
>
> *So, Anna spoke up and she said, Yeah, it's always negative, because I'm not a very good kid.*
>
> *I said, So tell me about that. Why do you think you're not good?*

*Anna replied, Because I think if I weren't here, my mommy and my daddy probably would have got along a lot better.*

*I said, Okay, can you tell me more about that?*

*Well, my mommy and daddy would often argue, and they'd say that their problems started when she got pregnant with me.*

*I asked Anna, Okay. Do you think that's true?*

*She said, Well, that's what they said.*

*So, she went on, and kept talking in the conversation and the mother, you know, you could tell by the lack of expression on her face that she really wasn't wanting Anna to tell this kind of stuff. So I said, Well, Anna, I don't think you have to tell me all the details, but what do you think you would like from me today? You don't know me very well, but what would you like from me today?*

*Anna said, Well, I think I need a hug.*

*So, she walked right over, and she hugged me, and it was such a hug. I thought, does this child get this* ***ever****? [Dr. Mary tears up.] So, the mother didn't respond much.*

*I said, Well, Anna, you know I do a little thing called Reiki. And so, I'm just kind of wondering if you and your mommy would be open to doing a little Reiki today. We don't have to talk much, but what Reiki does is it really relaxes people. It really helps the energy change in the room, and it really helps us kind of be present with each other. So do you think you might want to try that today?*

*Anna's mother said, Well, what is this?*

*I explained, It's just an energetic modality that I use a lot to kind of calm children who've been through a lot of trauma. It doesn't do anything to them except center them. And I'm not going to promise you anything, but we'll just see how Anna responds today.*

*Her mother said, Well, I don't want her doing this by herself.*

*I said, Nope. We're going to get you both up on the massage table here together, okay?*

*Anna's mother said, Well, can I stop this if I don't like it?*

*And I said, Absolutely.*

*She said, Is this going to make me start saying things I don't want to say?*

*I said, No, most of the time, this is very silent work.*

*So of course, in all of my rooms, you know we use aromatherapy, and we have soft music, so I really focused on that, and I got them both up there. Anna was very open to it from the beginning. You could just see how she was opening her heart. So, I just started from the top, and we just did an unruffling and we just kind of worked through it. And she was very comfortable from the start, closing her eyes. Her mother—it took her a while. So, by the time I did an energetic assessment, there was so much lack of energy flow—it was all in the center in the root Chakra so I could tell how much trauma had been there. So, I just worked on them for probably about an hour and they fell asleep. I let them sleep until they woke—it took about 45 minutes. So, I just stepped outside of the room and got some other stuff done and silently checked them a couple of times and then they both kind of woke up.*

*The mother was just like How long have we been here?*

*I said, Only a short time, about 45 minutes.*

*She said, Well, I really hadn't planned on staying that long.*

*I replied, Well, it's okay, you know there's nothing going on here that we need to hurry.*

*So, she said, Wow! I've never had anything like this before.*

*And I said, Well, I think most people probably haven't slowed down enough to feel this kind of experience, but I was happy to do that for you. Now what I'd like to do is to do some follow-up visits with you, because I think we need to work a little bit with Anna and maybe a lot with you. Where we can kind of—like peeling an onion, you just take the layers back. But I need you to know that I don't think Anna is a bad child at all. So, I want her to leave today not hearing that word again. She's very intuitive; she's very energetic. And we're going to start working to really help her move through what she's been through and most of all, what you've been through. So, what do you think about that?*

*And the mother's tears came to her eyes, and she said, You know, Mary, I just feel like you are a kindred spirit—like you maybe know what I'm going through without me telling you. And that I've never trusted anybody in quite the way I trust you today. I really do want to start working with you. I want Anna to see you.*

*And so, we did. I've seen her since she was seven. She's now 11 and she's going into middle school. She's just doing awesome. Was she constipated? No, she was traumatized. Was she anxious? Of course, she was anxious. She was coming into a stranger's room.*

*You know I've learned from Anna, I learned from her mother, but I learned from many other children. Many I worked with on the pain team at children's hospital were in so much pain, but if you could just sit there with them for a little bit and energetically change that environment and let them know they were loved and cared for, that really changes the whole perspective. And then you can do whatever it is you need to do, but you first have to let the child know that you care about them.*

*Anna contacted me the other day because her family is going to move back to [the Northeast] probably in the spring and she said that for the first time she's going to get to see her grandma in five years. And I said what a wonderful thing! And we talked a little bit about me being a grandma and what that means. But I think that family has been healed enough, you know? I talked to the mother a lot about where the partner is and he's left there, so hopefully this will all be positive for her.* (Hines, personal communication, December 10, 2021)

# Exploring the Emergence of the Holistic Healing Environment Framework

## Through and Within the Reflective Reflexive Process

Let's now explore the emergence of the HHE Framework through and within the reflective reflexive process in the Nursing Situation *I Trust You.* The reflective reflexive process is manifested within mutual process and *knowingdoingbecoming* from which emerges authentic presence, integral presence, and compassionate unity transcending suffering towards healing.

### Authentic Presence

How does Dr. Mary live authentic presence? Reflect on when the Nurses said, *"This is going to be just a horrible night" and her response to them: "Okay, let's all kind of come up here to the desk. We're going to get into a caring circle here and we're going to talk about this, because this is not how we're going to do this night. These patients are critically ill, and they need you to be present with them. They don't need you to bring in your stuff, okay? So, let's all kind of refocus here"* (Hines, personal communication, December 10, 2021).

### Integral Presence

Through *knowingdoingbecoming,* Dr. Mary becomes integrally present through perceiving-experiencing the integrality of herself as Nurse and environment—the wholeness of self and the interconnectedness of self with her patient. In her *knowingdoingbecoming, "You know energetically this room is tense to me. Are you guys feeling that?"* (Hines, personal communication, December 10, 2021).

### Compassionate Unity

She then emerges from integral presence to compassionate unity through and within the alternating rhythms of perceiving-experiencing *I feel you, you feel me, and I feel you feeling me* (Hübl, 2021, p. 2)—the interwoven energy field of herself as Nurse, her patient, and the patient's mother, simultaneously the healer and healee, all healing and all being healed. Within the HHE Framework, Dr. Mary comes to know the patient's call for love and acceptance.

> *"So, I said, 'Well, Anna, ... what do you think you would like from me today? You don't know me very well, but what would you like from me today'"?*
>
> *"Anna said, 'Well, I think I need a hug.'"*
>
> *"So, she walked right over, and she hugged me, and it was such a hug. I thought does this child get this* ***ever****?" [Dr. Mary tears up.]* (Hines, personal communication, December 10, 2021).

The call for Nursing in *any* Nursing Situation is experienced only through compassionate unity, which emerges through mutual process, knowing participation, and *knowingdoingbecoming.* Within compassionate unity, Dr. Mary co-creates a safe, holistic healing environment with aromatherapy and soft music as she intentionally does a holistic energy assessment and Reiki with Anna and her mother. They fell asleep awakening with peacefulness, calm, and ease from suffering finding meaning in the living experience.

> *"And the mother's tears came to her eyes, and she said, 'You know, Mary I just feel like you are a kindred spirit—like you maybe know what I'm going through without me telling you. And that I've never trusted anybody in quite the way I trust you today. I really do want to start working with you. I want Anna to see you'"* (Hines, personal communication, December 10, 2021).

Dr. Mary as Nurse is soul whisperer and healer.

## Summary

In this chapter, the practice of a holistic Nurse in a primary care setting is illuminated through the interpretation of the HHE Framework. Dr. Mary shared her personal perspective of what she considers key for Nurse in co-creating a holistic healing environment.

> *So, you've got to pay attention to the environment. But I think that's the part of who we are as Nurses—each one of us can walk into a room and because we are who we are, we can start the conversation, we can relax the patient. We can be present with them, and I think we're very open to cues of patients, and that's all part of that healing process: your intentionality, your caring consciousness, and most importantly, you've got to let go of everything before you enter that room. So, I say pause to care. You've got to pause for a minute. You've got to center yourself because every situation is going to be unique and different. And if you bring a whole bunch of energy and negativity into a situation, that's how it'll turn out."* (Hines, personal communication, December 10, 2021)

Through the Nursing Situation *"I trust you,"* we experience the emergence of compassionate unity within Dr. Mary's integral presence and the alternating rhythms of perceiving-experiencing *I feel you, you feel me, and I feel you feeling me* (Hübl, 2021, p. 2)—the interwoven energy field of Dr. Mary, her patient, and her patient's mother, all simultaneously the healer and healee, all healing and all being healed. Within compassionate unity, Dr. Mary as Nurse is soul whisperer and healer. This Nursing Situation is an exemplar of the dance of alternating rhythms with intentional knowing participation to co-create an environment through which holistic healing emerges for Nurse and person(s).

## Key Takeaways from This Chapter

Within this chapter, the Nurse's living experience of co-creating a holistic healing environment is revealed through the interpretation of the HHE Framework. Below is a list of key information and ideas to take away from your reading supported by Dr. Mary's own words (Hines, personal communication, December 10, 2021).

- Centering prepares the Nurse to be authentically present. *"You've got to pause for a minute. You've got to center yourself, because every situation is going to be unique and different. And if you bring a whole bunch of energy and negativity into a situation, that's how it'll turn out."*
- The Nurse as soul whisperer and healer can *"really shift the environment ... and open possibilities,"* which is the essence of co-creating a holistic healing environment.

## End-of-Chapter Questions, Applications, and Group Activities

**Directions:** Use what you have learned in this chapter to reflect upon and respond to the questions, applications, and group activities below.

## Questions

- Reflect on Dr. Mary's descriptions of entering the environment in a PICU and primary care setting. Identify the key elements that apply to all practice settings.

## Applications

- Dr. Mary shared, *"I experience healing every day with the smiles on those children's faces and the hugs they give me."* Reflect on how you experience healing every day.
- Reread what Anna's mother shared with Dr. Mary after experiencing Reiki—specifically trust. How does that resonate with you and your own feelings about trust between patient and Nurse, Nurse and Nurse, Nurse and other? Do you trust others? How is that manifested?

## Group Activities

- Which caring theory of Nursing do you see as guiding Dr. Mary in her practice? Why?
- Practice leading and participating in a caring circle. We have provided an example below but encourage you to create a caring circle with language you are comfortable with.

1. Gather persons in a circle, shoulder-to-shoulder.
2. Invite them to close or lower eyes as you lead them in an awareness exercise.
3. Focus on your breathing into your heart and out through your heart. Find a rhythm that is most comfortable for you.
4. As you continue to breathe in and out through your heart, image a place where you feel safe, feel joy, or feel gratitude. Actually feel this emotion in your heart.
5. As you continue to breathe in and out of your heart, bring that emotion with you as you return to this time and space.
6. Invite everyone to turn to their right, placing their hands on the shoulder of the person in front of them and offering a massage of the shoulders. With their hands, gently say goodbye to this person (gentle tapping on the shoulders).
7. Then turn to your left and give back what you've just received, placing their hands on the shoulder of the person in front of them and offering a massage of the shoulders. With their hands, gently say goodbye to this person (gentle tapping on the shoulders).
8. Invite everyone to face the inner circle and ask if anyone has something to say/offer to start the day.

5

# Peacefulness and Calm

## Introduction

In this chapter, we introduce you to Ms. Rose Hosler, BSN, RN, HNB-BC, HWNC-BC. She is board certified as a Holistic Nurse and Nurse Coach, certified in acupressure and clinical aromatherapy and is also a Reiki master. Her vast experience in surgical intensive care, emergency department, post-anesthesia care unit, and private duty have served her well as she has integrated holistic practice in her journey. For the past ten years, she has been practicing as a holistic Nurse in a 500-bed acute care hospital, seeing patients, families, and staff. Nurse Hosler speaks locally and nationally on holistic Nursing, integrative health, and stress management, and she works with staff and the community in crisis intervention. As a holistic Nurse she receives referrals from physicians, Nurses, and social workers to see patients for a variety of situations/reasons.

> *From a holistic perspective, it is great in that I have a strong clinical foundation so that I can really understand what's going on with someone clinically. As I'm in this role, specifically as a holistic Nurse, I can really integrate and see the larger picture for someone and really look at within that context of a holistic framework. And then of course I'm able to use many different tools, depending on what the situation is for, and so that's where I can bring in some holistic modalities if needed. So, when I meet with someone, I introduce myself as a holistic Nurse. And I always ask, "May I pull up a chair," and more often than not the answer is "please do.'"* (R. Hosler, personal communication, November 8, 2021)

Hosler receives referrals through electronic health record (EHR) as well as verbally from physicians, Nurses, other members of the healthcare team, and patients themselves. *"When I receive a referral, my role is I travel throughout the hospital, so I am not specific to one unit or department." She emphasized the importance of how she gets to go to so many different departments in the acute care setting, but how she is also involved with the community teaching about stress, [wellbecoming] and holistic care. "In this role, I can get referrals to see patients for anything, but I would say the top things are pain, emotional support, anxiety, and/or a new difficult diagnosis. And to help someone with relaxation—that kind of goes hand in hand with pain at times"* (R. Hosler, personal communication, November 8, 2021). Hosler shared that she could be called into the delivery room or surgery to be with the patient and family or to a unit "to help a Nurse who may be experiencing a meltdown" (R. Hosler, personal communication, November 8, 2021).

We asked Nurse Hosler, from her perspective, what is an essential element for co-creating a holistic healing environment in practice. *"While I am walking to another patient room, I am mindful, and do focused breathing. When called to see a Nurse or other staff member for support, I do center and ground. I do set an intention and say a prayer prior to going out on the units"* (R. Hosler, personal communication, November 8, 2021).

She expanded upon what is essential: *"So, for me, I would say, being present with the patient, and I have no expectation with the patient. And I think that really contributes to co-creating the healing environment. I always introduce myself and I let the patient take the lead, so I'm present with them. It's okay if they say no, if they choose that they really don't want to talk with me or sit with me or anything like that. So, I don't need anything from them, I don't need to get their vitals, I don't need to go into a long conversation with them"* (R. Hosler, personal communication, November 8, 2021).

**Thoughtful Reflections**

Reflect upon "*being present and having no expectations.*" Reframe this within authentic presence.

### Objectives

After completing this chapter, readers will:

- Within the Nurse's living experience described in this chapter, identify the patterns of knowing and ingredients of caring.
- Within the HHE Framework, describe the Nurse's *knowingdoingbecoming* as soul whisperer and healer in the context of the Nursing Situation described above.
- Demonstrate the reflective reflexive process in applying the HHE Framework within the selected Nursing Situation.

### Key Terms and Concepts

**Directions:** Before continuing, we encourage you to take time to refamiliarize yourself with key concepts from Chapter 4 that are integral to understanding Nurses' living experience in co-creating a holistic healing environment.

## Nursing Situation: *Peacefulness and Calm*

We asked Nurse Hosler to share a Nursing Situation in which she co-created an environment that supported healing not only for the patient but for his sons and her as well.

> *I had a patient who was in the ICU (intensive care unit) and he had been really struggling. He happened to be in the bed that actually folds up into a chair, so they could put him in a sitting*

*position when I had been working with him. And then one day, when I was in there and as we were talking, he said that he just needed to feel some peacefulness and some calmness. And as we all know, in the ICUs, it's a very intense place to be—monitors and the beeping and all the in-and-out and everything that's happening. And his sons happened to be visiting that day. And he wanted to experience Reiki. His sons were going to stay in the room during the session, which he asked for. He wanted Reiki. I always ask for permission to touch or not to touch, depending on their preference, and he did not want to be touched. So, I began the Reiki session, and about two to three minutes into it, you could just see it in his face as he became relaxed, and he just had this look of peacefulness over him. And, at the end of the session—we went about 15 minutes—he opened his eyes and he said, "I haven't felt that peacefulness definitely since I've been in the hospital, but I can't tell you the last time I even felt that sense of peacefulness in my life." And the sons were just sitting there, and they were also calm, and they were amazed at how calm and peaceful their dad was. And so, it created that space just for the quietness for him to receive, and I think it gave his sons an opportunity to see their dad in a peaceful state and calm amongst this kind of intense at times chaotic intensive care unit—you know, there is not much peace in an ICU unit. And so, I think for me that the healing was being able to be in this space with someone and support what they needed at that time. And so, I think that supported my own healing experience. I think that even the sons experienced healing, as they were in that environment as a whole family unit, and they experienced this together; even though they weren't getting Reiki, they were in that time and space, which was wonderful. (R. Hosler, personal communication, November 8, 2021).*

**Thoughtful Reflection**

Within this Nursing Situation, reflect on Nurse Hosler as soul whisperer and healer.

# Exploring the Emergence of the Holistic Healing Environment Framework

## Through and Within the Reflective Reflexive Process

Let's now explore the emergence of the HHE Framework through and within the reflective reflexive process in the Nursing Situation *Peacefulness and Calm.* The reflective reflexive process is manifested within mutual process and *knowingdoingbecoming* from which emerges authentic presence, integral presence, and compassionate unity transcending suffering towards healing.

### *Authentic Presence*

How does Nurse Hosler live authentic presence? She began by sharing how she prepares herself to enter a patient's room or when called to support a Nurse or other staff member using the techniques of mindfulness, focused breathing, prayer, grounding, and centering. Grounding and centering are foundational in caring for self and preparing self to be authentically present. Within the HHE Framework, exemplars of these techniques also include heart-focused breathing, meditation, and/or imagery.

### *Integral Presence*

Through *knowingdoingbecoming,* she becomes integrally present through perceiving-experiencing the integrality of herself as Nurse and environment—the wholeness of self and the interconnectedness of self with her patient. In her *knowingdoingbecoming,* she knew how her patient was struggling: *"I had a patient who was in the ICU, and he had been really struggling."*

### *Compassionate Unity*

She then emerges from integral presence to compassionate unity through and within the alternating rhythms of perceiving-experiencing *I feel you, you feel me, and I feel you feeling me* (Hübl, 2021, p. 2)—the interwoven energy field of herself as Nurse and her patient, simultaneously the healer and healee, both healing and both being healed. Within the HHE Framework, Nurse Hosler comes to know her patient's call for peace: *"He just needed to feel some peacefulness and some calmness."* The call for Nursing in *any* Nursing Situation is experienced only through compassionate unity, which emerges through mutual process, knowing participation, and *knowingdoingbecoming.*

Within compassionate unity, Nurse Hosler co-designs holistic Nursing care with her patient as she mindfully and critically evaluates and integrates Reiki to assure safe, holistic healing, helping her patient to find meaning in the living experience manifested as peacefulness, calm, and transcending suffering. She asks her patient if he wanted touch or no touch, respecting his dignity and honoring his choice. *"And, at the end of the session—we went about 15 minutes—he opened his eyes and he said, 'I haven't felt that peacefulness since I've been in the hospital, but I can't tell you the last time I even felt that sense of peacefulness in my life."*

As Nurse Hosler and her patient's environment also included his sons, as an energy therapy the peacefulness and calm experienced within Reiki simultaneously benefited Nurse Hosler, her patient, and his sons in assisting with healing (Brathovde, 2017). *"And the sons were just sitting there, and they were also calm, and they were amazed at how calm and peaceful their dad was."*

> *"... I think for me that the healing was being able to be in this space with someone and support what they needed at that time. And so, I think that supported my own healing experience. I think that even the sons experienced healing as they were in that environment as a whole family unit and they experienced this together; even though they weren't getting Reiki, they were in in that time and space, which was wonderful."* (R. Hosler, personal communication, November 8, 2021)

## Summary

In this chapter, the practice of a holistic Nurse in an acute care setting is illuminated through the interpretation of the HHE Framework. Nurse Hosler shares her personal perspective of what she considers key in co-creating a holistic healing environment—integral presence and having no expectations from the patient and/or family. Through the Nursing Situation, we experience the emergence of compassionate unity within Nurse Hosler's integral presence and the alternating rhythms of perceiving-experiencing *I feel you, you feel me, and I feel you feeling me* (Hübl, 2021, p. 2)—the interwoven energy field of Nurse Hosler and her patient and his sons, all simultaneously the healer and healee, all healing and all being healed. Within compassionate unity, Nurse Hosler is soul whisperer and healer. This Nursing Situation is an exemplar of the dance of alternating rhythms with intentional knowing participation to co-create an environment through which holistic healing emerges for Nurse and person(s).

## Key Takeaways from This Chapter

Within this chapter, the Nurse's living experience of co-creating a holistic healing environment is revealed through the interpretation of the HHE Framework. Below is a list of key information and ideas to take away from your reading supported by Nurse Hosler's own words (R. Hosler, personal communication, November 8, 2021).

- The emergence of the HHE Framework is explored through and within the reflective reflexive process in this Nursing Situation.
- The reflective reflexive process is manifested within mutual process and *knowingdoingbecoming,* from which emerges authentic presence, integral presence, and compassionate unity transcending suffering towards healing.
- Grounding and centering are foundational in caring for self and preparing self to be authentically present.
- Within compassionate unity, the interwoven energy field of Nurse as soul whisperer, patient, and family experience simultaneous healing, all healing, and all being healed.

## End-of-Chapter Questions, Applications, and Group Activities

**Directions:** Use what you have learned in this chapter to reflect upon and respond to the questions, applications, and group activities below.

### Questions

- When did Nurse Hosler manifest authentic presence, integral presence, and compassionate unity?
- How did the Nurse, patient, and family experience healing in the Nursing Situation *Peacefulness and Calm*?

## Applications

- Within the HHE Framework, identify and describe exemplars of Nurse Hosler's *knowingdoingbecoming.*
- Every Nursing Situation is open to emerging possibilities. Within this context, what might you have done that reflects your *knowingdoingbecoming*?
- As grounding and centering are foundational in caring for self and preparing self to be authentically present, select a grounding and centering approach that resonates with you to apply in your practice.

## Group Activities

- Which caring theory of Nursing do you see as guiding Nurse Hosler in her practice? Why?
- Nurse Hosler holds a unique position in this hospital as a dedicated holistic Nurse. What might care look like in this or any hospital if all Nurses practiced within the HHE Framework?

6

# "150 Miles an Hour"

## Introduction

Let us introduce you to Nurse Marcie Resnicoff, BSN, BS, RN, HNB-BC, the clinical Nurse coordinator in a hospital-based health promotion-integrative health department in the northeast. Nurse Resnicoff is a board-certified Holistic Nurse and has a certificate in holistic nutrition. She is a Reiki master practitioner and teacher and has taught mindfulness, guided imagery, and other forms of meditation, wellness, Reiki, and self-care. She has more than 20 years of experience using mind-body therapies and has more than a decade of patient care Nursing experience at the same hospital. She is currently pursuing her master's degree in advanced holistic Nursing.

Nurse Resnicoff did not grow up wanting to be a Nurse but was called to Nursing later in her life.

> *I'm a late-in-life Nurse. I've only been a Nurse since 2008 and I've been in the same hospital the whole time. But the hospital system changed and like so many others, it was taken over, so now we're part of this larger enterprise which changes things up, but it also affords us so much more access to really high-quality, innovative care, which is really a plus. So, before Nursing—and this is important because it's what brought me to Nursing—I was an actor and I primarily did theater and improv theater. Because I eked out a living, I was really poor, and I couldn't really afford health insurance. So, I spent a lot of my time trying to avoid needing to go to the doctor. I only went when I was really, really sick. And instead, I learned a whole bunch of tools that I could use to help me stay well. So, I became a Reiki practitioner, and I started meditating and I really started studying nutrition on my own to learn how I can use nutrition to stay healthier. And over the course of time, I just became really passionate about it, and I had no idea that there was a holistic Nursing organization. I was a very Western medicine girl, so this was all new to me. And I remember thinking, I'd really like to become a Nurse, so I can bridge Eastern and Western medicine, because more people need to know how to do this.*
>
> *So, I became a Nurse, and you know it was slow going at first, in that I started off in medsurg. I did my night shift; I did the day shift; I started off working surgery trauma; and then I was trained in this step-down unit for surgery trauma. So, I did that for a number of years, and then I was asked to move to rehab to start incorporating some of my holistic tools with patients who were there for two weeks at a time, sometimes longer. I started doing that work and when [another system] took over ownership of my old hospital, it came with a gift agreement to create an integrative health*

> *department in my hospital, and they asked me to be one of the people to help develop it. So that's how I got to be in integrative health and really go full circle back to my original plan.* (Resnicoff, personal communication, November 15, 2021).

Nurse Resnicoff shared that she experiences healing through the joy of connecting fully with another.

> *Anytime that I'm able to connect fully with another person, that I could be grounded enough and present enough to really feel a heart-to-heart connection with them, it always brings me a moment of joy. And so, even the hardest moment of the day has those moments of joy in it, because it reminds me, I'm taking care of my family right now, this is my work family. It's very healing for me to get the feedback of knowing that I was able to be present for somebody in a healthy way.* (Resnicoff, personal communication, November 15, 2021)

We asked Nurse Resnicoff, from her perspective, what is an essential element for co-creating a holistic healing environment in practice. In her perception and words, she describes being authentically present.

> For me, I think it's really important that I'm completely present and grounded. Because if I'm anxious, I sometimes feel like I've disconnected—my body is here, and my spirit's over there, my brain is there, and so, if I'm grounded and present, I'm better able to connect with others, whether I'm doing a class where I'm teaching a whole presentation, or whether I'm doing a one-on-one. ... My goal with this is always to offer myself as a caring presence for one person ... or a whole unit. (Resnicoff, personal communication, November 15, 2021)

**Thoughtful Reflections**

Reflect upon Nurse Resnicoff's understanding of healing within the importance of *heart-to-heart connection and experiencing moments of joy even during the hardest moments of the day*. How does this idea resonate within your practice?

### Objectives

After completing this chapter, readers will:

- Within the Nurse's living experience described in this chapter, identify the patterns of knowing and ingredients of caring.
- Within the HHE Framework, describe the Nurse's *knowingdoingbecoming* as soul whisperer and healer in the context of the Nursing Situation "150 Miles an Hour".
- Demonstrate the reflective reflexive process in applying the HHE Framework within the selected Nursing Situation.

**Key Terms and Concepts**

**Directions:** Before continuing, we encourage you to take time to become familiar with key concepts.

- **Integrative health**—Partnering with person in his/her wholeness to support wellbecoming and find meaning in the health experience through reflection, identification of patterns, and opportunities for healing.
- **Integrative healthcare**—Nurse, person, family, and interprofessional team co-coordinate conventional and complementary approaches for healing.
- **Holism**—A pandimensional view of person in his/her wholeness, lifeworld, and being.
- **Holistic**—Greater than and different from the sum of parts.
- **Wholeness**—*Heartmindbodysoul.*

## Nursing Situation: *"150 Miles an Hour"*

Nurse Resnicoff shared the following Nursing Situation. It is an exemplar of how every moment is different—whether it's person-to-person or unit-to-unit, reminding the Nurse to pause, ground, and center to become authentically present to influence the environment.

> *Since the pandemic, the work I do has changed. In the beginning, it was going to be probably 50:50 working with staff, teaching them tools, doing a train-the-trainer, and then working with patients half the time. And now it's like at least 80% staff. And so, the work that I do and the work that my colleague, the program manager, does ... we are developing programs and classes mostly for the staff to incorporate self-care into their days, and I hope, with the belief that if we take care of them, if they feel supported, if they feel cared for, if they feel like their cup is being replenished a little bit, then the patients will be better taken care of.*
>
> *And so, one program since the pandemic and pre-vaccine that I was asked to be involved with is to help develop a peer-to-peer group, and this was an interdisciplinary project. We had a couple of psychiatrists and chaplains involved. We had Nurse managers, Nursing directors, and then also some clinical Nurses that were involved in putting this together. So, one of the things that we felt had to happen is a peer-to-peer response because a lot of the staff didn't have time to process the first wave of the pandemic. And then we were in a lull and suddenly the second wave was coming, but they were always so busy just catching up with whatever they were doing, so we developed this program.*
>
> *Some of us volunteered to be trained in mental health first aid and motivational interviewing. It's not that I have more time than everybody else, but I made it part of what I do. So at least once a week I'm walking through the hospital units or checking on people that I meet in the hallway, or you know, wherever I see them and checking in and seeing how they're doing and really holding*

*space for them. Sometimes I'm sharing self-care tools, sometimes I'm just listening, sometimes I am offering self-care goodies—like we have these lavender tabs of aromatherapy that they could take home and put on their pillows to help them sleep at night. And we also have acupressure ear seeds that go on; we have instructions that they go on a stress spot on the ear, and they can use those to help just calm their fight or flight mechanism. My goal with this is always to offer myself as a caring presence for either one person or sometimes working with a whole unit. And I try to make sure that I've succeeded in making sure that people know that I'm a trustworthy person that they could speak to if they are having trouble.*

*There was a situation where there was a high stress event on a unit. Psychiatry was called and I was called. And so, in this situation, the Nurse manager said to me, "We'll huddle with everyone together at this time, but could you first go check on this Nurse for me?" So, I went and the one specific Nurse that I checked on was actually the charge Nurse, and she was like, "No, no, I'm fine. I'm good. I just I have a lot to do. I have to catch up on the meds and I have to do this, you know, because that event happened."*

*And I said, "You know what? You need a minute."*

*She was going at 150 miles an hour; she was running on adrenaline; she didn't feel very grounded; she was just in her to-do list mode. So, I took her to a quiet empty room on the unit, and I said, "I get you for five minutes. That's all it takes—five minutes."*

*And I brought her in, and I said, "I need to check on you, because I'm sensing that this was very emotional for you, and you're not really feeling grounded right now. And I don't want that to carry on throughout your day."*

*So, I started. She allowed me to give her some Reiki while she was telling me her story, and then I did a grounded-focused breathing technique with her to slow down her breathing and help her reset herself. And just to notice the wave of relaxation and calm come over her and she even noticed it. She said, "Oh, I guess, I really did need that."*

*The Nurse was able to feel a lot more grounded and calm, and so she could really go back to her being present and caring for others.* (Resnicoff, personal communication, November 15, 2021)

# Exploring the Emergence of the Holistic Healing Environment Framework

## Through and Within the Reflective Reflexive Process

Let's now explore the emergence of the HHE Framework through and within the reflective reflexive process in the Nursing Situation *"150 Miles an Hour"*. The reflective reflexive process is manifested within mutual process and *knowingdoingbecoming* from which emerges authentic presence, integral presence, and compassionate unity transcending suffering towards healing.

### *Authentic Presence*

How does Nurse Resnicoff prepare self for and live authentic presence? Reflect on her words for preparing self:

> *For me, I think it's really important that I'm completely present and grounded. Because if I'm anxious, I sometimes feel like I've disconnected—my body is here, and my spirit's over there, my brain is there, and so, if I'm grounded and present, I'm better able to connect with others.* (Resnicoff, personal communication, November 15, 2021)

This illuminates Nurse Resnicoff's awareness of and coming-to-know self in synchrony and harmony within alternating rhythms guided by Mayeroff's ingredients of caring and Roach's caring attributes to choose *who I bring to practice in this moment.*

Who she *chooses to bring to practice in this moment* is then manifested as authentic presence when she shared:

> *I'm walking through the hospital units or checking on people that I meet in the hallway, or you know, wherever I see them and checking in and seeing how they're doing and really holding space for them. My goal with this is always to offer myself as a caring presence for either one person or sometimes working with a whole unit.* (Resnicoff, personal communication, November 15, 2021)

### *Integral Presence*

Through *knowingdoingbecoming,* she becomes integrally present through perceiving-experiencing the integrality of herself as Nurse and environment—the wholeness of self and the interconnectedness of self with her peer, the charge Nurse. In her *knowingdoingbecoming,* integral presence is manifested within *"And I said, 'you know what? You need a minute'"* (Resnicoff, personal communication, November 15, 2021).

### *Compassionate Unity*

She then emerges from integral presence to compassionate unity through and within the alternating rhythms of perceiving-experiencing *I feel you, you feel me, and I feel you feeling me* (Hübl, 2021, p. 2)—the interwoven energy field of herself as Nurse and her patient (the charge Nurse), simultaneously the healer and healee, both healing and both being healed. Within the HHE Framework, Nurse Resnicoff comes to know the charge Nurse's call for slowing down.

> *She was going at 150 miles an hour; she was running on adrenaline; she didn't feel very grounded; she was just in her to-do list mode. And I said, "I need to check on you, because I'm sensing that this was very emotional for you, and you're not really feeling grounded right now. And I don't want that to carry on throughout your day." She allowed me to give her some Reiki while she was telling me her story, and then I did a grounded-focused breathing technique with her to slow down her breathing and help her reset herself. And just to notice the wave of relaxation and calm come over her, and she even noticed it. She said, "Oh, I guess, I really did need that."* (Resnicoff, personal communication, November 15, 2021)

The call for Nursing in *any* Nursing Situation is experienced only through compassionate unity, which emerges through mutual process, knowing participation, and *knowingdoingbecoming.* Within compassionate unity, Nurse Resnicoff co-created a safe, holistic healing environment in a quiet empty room on the unit assuring the charge Nurse to trust that she only needed five minutes. In those five minutes, she performed Reiki and used *"a grounded focused breathing technique with her to slow down her breathing"* within which they simultaneously experienced relaxation and calm. The charge Nurse experienced ease from suffering the emotional impact from the high stress event on the unit finding meaning in the living experience. *She said, "Oh, I guess, I really did need that."*

> *"The Nurse was able to feel a lot more grounded and calm, and so she could really go back to her being present and caring for others"* (Resnicoff, personal communication, November 15, 2021).

Nurse Resnicoff is soul whisperer and healer.

## Summary

In this chapter, the practice of a holistic Nurse as the clinical Nurse coordinator at a hospital-based health promotion-integrative health department in the northeast is illuminated through the interpretation of the HHE Framework. Nurse Resnicoff shared her personal perspective of what she considers key for Nurse in co-creating a holistic healing environment. She emphasized that as every moment is different (person-to-person, unit-to-unit), the Nurse must pause, ground, and center to become authentically present to emerge to integral presence to then experience the *heart-to-heart connection* of compassionate unity. Since the pandemic, her practice has shifted to mainly working with Nurses and staff *"with the belief that if we take care of them, if they feel supported, if they feel cared for, if they feel like their cup is being replenished a little bit, then the patients will be better taken care of."*

Through the Nursing Situation *"150 Miles an Hour,"* we experience the emergence of compassionate unity within Nurse Resnicoff's integral presence and the alternating rhythms of perceiving-experiencing *I feel you, you feel me, and I feel you feeling me* (Hübl, 2021, p. 2)—the interwoven energy field of Nurse Resnicoff and the charge Nurse, both simultaneously the healer and healee, both healing and both being healed. Within compassionate unity, Nurse Resnicoff is soul whisperer and healer. This Nursing Situation is an exemplar of the dance of alternating rhythms with intentional knowing participation to co-create an environment through which holistic healing emerges for Nurse and person(s).

## Key Takeaways from This Chapter

Within this chapter, the Nurse's living experience of co-creating a holistic healing environment is revealed through the interpretation of the HHE Framework. Below is a list of key information and ideas to take away from your reading, supported by Nurse Resnicoff's own words (Resnicoff, personal communication, November 15, 2021).

- *"Every moment is different—person-to-person, unit-to-unit."*
- Within integrative health, we partner with a person in his/her wholeness to support wellbecoming and find meaning in the health experience through reflection, identification of patterns, and opportunities for healing.
- When the Nurse as soul whisperer and healer co-creates a holistic healing environment, Nurses and staff feel supported and cared for—*"like their cup is being replenished a little bit, then the patients will be better taken care of"* (Resnicoff, personal communication, November 15, 2021).
- It is important to remember that Nurse can co-create a holistic healing environment in a few minutes. *"That's all it takes—five minutes."*

## End-of-Chapter Questions, Applications, and Group Activities

**Directions:** Use what you have learned in this chapter to reflect upon and respond to the questions, applications, and group activities below.

### Questions and Reflection

- Reflect on Nurse Resnicoff's description of *"the belief that if we take care of [Nurses, staff], if they feel supported, if they feel cared for, if they feel like their cup is being replenished a little bit, then the patients will be better taken care of."* How is the reflective reflexive process manifested within mutual process and *knowingdoingbecoming* from which emerges a co-created holistic healing environment within which suffering is transcended through and within healing?

### Applications

- Nurse Resnicoff shared that she *"experiences moments of joy even during the hardest moments of the day."* Reflect on how you experience moments of joy during moments of your practice.

### Group Activities

- Which caring theory of Nursing do you see as guiding Nurse Resnicoff in her practice? Why?
- Nurse Resnicoff was recruited to help develop an integrative health department. How would you co-create an integrative health department in your facility, and how would you garner support for its development?

# 7

# Struggling to Walk the Walk

## Introduction

In this chapter, we introduce you to Nurse Courtny Hopen, BSN, RN, CMS-RN, HNB-BC. Nurse Hopen is board-certified in two specialties: as a holistic Nurse and as a medical/surgical Nurse. She has extensive experience in medical/surgical Nursing with LGBTQ populations in New York City. Following graduation with a Bachelor of Science in Nursing (BSN) degree, she entered a Nurse residency program and conducted an evidence-based practice (EBP) project titled "*Beyond Pronouns: Interventions to Improve LGB and Transgender Patient Care.*"

> *They asked us to identify a population that needed some sort of intervention. And for me, it was very obvious, as on my floor, 12 East, we went from having approximately 20 patients who were having gender affirmation surgery to over 200 when the hospital hired a new surgeon who specialized in gender affirmation surgery. Most of the Nurses on our unit did not know how to take care of these patients. The two people who did know how to how to do it were me and this other Nurse, and we were the only LGBTQ Nurses. And we each had different experiences. I had a personal experience of taking care of someone in my life who had had gender affirmation surgery, so I knew about the different specialized procedures that you needed to do after surgery.* (Hopen, personal communication, December 1, 2021)

When asked what Nurse Hopen thought was important for Nurses to know to co-create a holistic healing environment for the transgender population, she stated:

> *So I think it's important to bring your whole self to your practice. Like what I've found is that my life experiences have enriched my ability to connect with patients, whether I know the patients or not. And I try to take care of the patient and treat their situation, as if the patient is my own relative or loved one. Like in my own experiences, where the healthcare system has failed me, they have given me inspiration for areas to improve on—both through things like the evidence-based practice project but also in areas of my own practice. If I feel myself getting caught up in like "Oh, I have to finish all these tasks" or like if I feel myself starting to get caught dehumanizing the patient and only thinking about what I need to do, I try to bring myself back to the present moment. I would use some mindfulness meditation and try to do like a little deep breathing and try to just be present with the patient.* (Hopen, personal communication, December 1, 2021)

**Thoughtful Reflections**

Reflect upon Nurse Hopen's statement about being authentically present: *"So I think it's important to bring your whole self to your practice."* How do you bring your whole self to your practice?

When reflecting upon what is an essential element for co-creating a holistic healing environment, Nurse Hopen offered two essential elements: teamwork and caring. She shared how they had an amazing team come together: the Nurse manager, assistant Nurse manager, assistant director for LGBTQ clinical services, Nurse Hopen, and her peer. *"We came together to talk about how we should educate the Nurses and make sure that this patient population gets the care that they need."* As a team, they co-created the Transgender Council on the unit. *"If we didn't have the support of different people who each had a stake in the patient getting better and with the patient themselves, ... co creating of healing wouldn't work"* (Hopen, personal communication, December 1, 2021).

The second essential element she identified was caring.

> *It comes back to Boykin and Schoenhofer with Nursing as caring because taking care of the patients, you have to actually care about their outcomes. One of the worst things that people do to them is they dehumanize them. There's a lot of transgender violence against transgender people. And one of the things that comes up over and over again in that violence is the perpetrators of the violence will call the transgender person an "It." They won't see them as the same kind of human that everyone else is. They will dehumanize them, and I think that the opposite of that is caring. Caring is the opposite of dehumanization. And I think that is just so essential to be caring about people as people. Not just did we meet our metric or what did they rate us, or what have you, but this person gets seen for the full human that they are. And they get treated with the same respect that everyone is deserving of.* (Hopen, personal communication, December 1, 2021)

Co-creating a holistic healing environment extended beyond the patients and Nurses to the loved ones. Nurse Hopen really enjoyed her practice as there was a teaching element involved. *"So, I felt like I was not only educating the other Nurses but also educating families and loved ones about their care. I felt like I was a particularly good fit because I had been on the other side of it. I had been a loved one of someone transgender who had been taught by a Nurse like six years before being on this unit."*

Nurse Hopen shared how reliving the experience of having respectful caring Nurses for her loved one was very meaningful to now be able to be on the other side of that experience. *"I'm going to be empowering these other loved ones. Everyone is going to work together to make this surgery a success and help the patient to feel more comfortable in their own skin, even though it's going to be an uncomfortable healing process"* (Hopen, personal communication, December 1, 2021).

Caring for self is also essential for *knowingdoingbecoming* within this practice.

> *I felt very blessed to have really good relationships with the other Nurses. So, to have time to decompress and to talk about what was going on with the other Nurses, sometimes after a long day we would go out to a diner and have pancakes. Because it's in New York City, you can get breakfast at any hour! I do yoga or go out dancing—do things that are full of joy.*

*Part of what has happened to me is like I'm a member of the LGBTQ community as well, and over the years I've had certain negative experiences with health care providers. To be on the front lines of changing that for other people was like very healing for me personally—to be like, oh, I don't ever want someone to have to go through what I went through. I want to try to be a positive change. That was very healing for me. Healing for the patients, I would say there were certain goals that we had to directly address, like the healthcare disparity that LGBTQ patients face, and try to affect that and change it. We were identifying Nursing knowledge gaps and remedying them through education. We were trying to increase Nursing staff confidence so that patients would experience having confident Nurses who were taking care of them. And then we are also trying to increase LGBTQ patient satisfaction scores, which is just like our measurable way of saying we want the patients to be having a better experience. Because I was very transparent about what we were doing on the unit about how we were addressing disparities and also had a Transgender Council that I was a member of, if they had any concerns or questions about it, they could bring them to me or to our managers who were also on the Council. I'm this person. I think we experienced a shared healing as fellow LGBTQ members.* (Hopen, personal communication, December 1, 2021)

**Thoughtful Reflections**

Reflect upon two essential elements of healing identified by Nurse Hopen: teamwork and caring. How do these elements resonate with your practice?

## Objectives

After completing this chapter, readers will:

- Within the Nurse's living experience described in this chapter, identify the patterns of knowing and ingredients of caring.
- Within the HHE Framework, describe the Nurse's *knowingdoingbecoming* as soul whisperer and healer in the context of the Nursing Situation Struggling to Walk the Walk.
- Demonstrate the reflective reflexive process in applying the HHE Framework within the selected Nursing Situation.

## Key Terms and Concepts

**Directions:** Before continuing, we encourage you to take time to become familiar with key concepts integral to understanding Nurses' living experience in co-creating a holistic healing environment.

- **Transgender**—"Designating a person whose sense of personal identity and gender does not correspond to that person's sex at birth, or which does not otherwise conform to conventional notions of sex and gender" (Simpson, Weiner, & Oxford University Press, 1988).

- **Gender affirmation surgery**—"Provides reconstructive care that centers your vision for aligning your body and anatomy to your gender identity" (NYU Langone Health, 2022).
- **Unknowing**—Choosing to be open in *heartmindbodysoul* to come to know other in the moment.

## Nursing Situation: *Struggling to Walk the Walk*

Nurse Hopen shared the following Nursing Situation:

> *There was actually a friend of mine who I had been out of touch with for a couple of years who showed up one day on our floor as a patient who had gotten gender affirmation surgery. I had been totally surprised. I had known this person when they identified as a woman, so I was used to using "she" and "her" pronouns. My whole conception of them was different from what they presented as, because they had had chest surgery and had their breasts removed. And they now use "they/them" pronouns, so I was like, all right, you know it's time for me to like walk the walk—this is their gender choice. I have to reconfigure my mind to make sure that I create a good healing environment and that I don't automatically slip up because I have this picture of them as their old self. And "they" were totally surprised. "They" were just like, "Hey, Courtny! So, you did end up going to Nursing school," and I was like, "I did." I tried not to let it become too much about the personal aspect because I wanted to make sure that they felt cared for medically. And so, I would be calm and professional and make sure that I was addressing all their medical concerns as opposed to chatting as old friends. It was interesting because, if they had used the name I had known them by, I would have requested not to be their Nurse because I would have felt like they should get someone who doesn't have past personal connection. But I was also like I'm probably the only person on the floor who is a member of the Transgender Council and they're probably going to get the best LGBTQ sensitive care from me that particular day.*
>
> *So, it was an interesting situation. At one point I actually did mis-gender that patient and I was like, I'm just going to do exactly what I tell everyone to do: just apologize and move on; don't make a big deal of it. I'd never had that happen before. As a member of Transgender Council who's doing all these services with the other Nurses, I felt like it helped build rapport that I messed up this person's pronouns. This is just what I did and instead of just lecturing people and being like, "You should do this" or "You should do that," people were like, "Oh Courtny is like walking the walk and like struggling too." And I felt like that actually built some more team unity on the floor.* (Hopen, personal communication, December 1, 2021)

# Exploring the Emergence of the Holistic Healing Environment Framework

## Through and Within the Reflective Reflexive Process

Let's now explore the emergence of the HHE Framework through and within the reflective reflexive process within her practice and the Nursing Situation *Struggling to Walk the Walk*. The reflective reflexive process is manifested within mutual process and *knowingdoingbecoming* from which emerges authentic presence, integral presence, and compassionate unity transcending suffering towards healing.

### *Authentic Presence*

How does Nurse Hopen live authentic presence? *"So, I think it's important to bring your whole self to your practice."* She emphasized the importance of caring for self, the importance of good relationships with the other Nurses on the unit, and doing things that are full of joy. Within the HHE Framework, reflect on how Nurse Hopen's living experience helped with *knowingdoingbecoming*.

### *Integral Presence*

Emerging from authentic presence to integral presence, Nurse Hopen's *knowingdoingbecoming* is further illuminated as she realizes she knows her patient. The reflective reflexive process begins unfolding here as she reflects on her past living experience with the patient, what her patient is currently experiencing, and then comes to know that she was meant to be her patient's Nurse that particular day. *"If I had used the name I had known them by, I would have requested not to be their Nurse because I would have felt like they should get someone who doesn't have that personal connection. But I was also like, I'm probably the only person on the floor who is a member of the Transgender Council and they're probably going to get the best LGBTQ sensitive care from me that particular day."* Nurse Hopen becomes integrally present through perceiving-experiencing the integrality of herself as Nurse and environment—the wholeness of self and the interconnectedness of self with her patient.

### *Compassionate Unity*

She then emerges from integral presence to compassionate unity through and within the alternating rhythms of perceiving-experiencing *I feel you, you feel me, and I feel you feeling me* (Hübl, 2021, p. 2)—the interwoven energy field of herself as Nurse and her patient, simultaneously the healer and healee, both healing and both being healed. Within the HHE Framework, Nurse Hopen comes to know the call for *unknowing*—choosing to be open in *heartmindbodysoul* to come to know other in the moment. *"My whole conception of them was different from what they presented as, because they had had chest surgery and had their breasts removed. And they now use 'they/them' pronouns. This is their gender choice. I have to reconfigure my mind to make sure that I create a good healing environment."* The call for Nursing in *any* Nursing Situation is experienced only through compassionate unity, which emerges through mutual process, knowing participation, and *knowingdoingbecoming*.

Within compassionate unity, Nurse Hopen co-created a holistic healing environment by suspending past personal knowing to open her *heartmindbodysoul* to help other transcend suffering towards healing and find meaning in the living experience through and within caring. *"I don't ever want someone to have to go through what I went through. I want to try to be a positive change"* (Hopen, personal communication, December 1, 2021).

Nurse Hopen is soul whisperer and healer.

## Summary

In this chapter, we explored Nurse Hopen's holistic practice with transgender persons undergoing gender affirmation surgery through an interpretation of the HHE Framework. From her perspective, the key for Nurse to co-create a holistic healing environment is to bring self in his/her wholeness to practice. Through her living experience and struggle in coming to know self, she intentionally chooses who she brings to practice.

> *Part of what has happened to me is like I'm a member of the LGBT community as well, and over the years I've had certain negative experiences with health care providers. To be on the front lines of changing that for other people was like very healing for me personally—to be like, oh I don't ever want someone to have to go through what I went through. I want to try to be a positive change.* (Hopen, personal communication, December 1, 2021)

## Key Takeaways from This Chapter

Within this chapter, the Nurse's living experience of co-creating a holistic healing environment is revealed through the interpretation of the HHE Framework. Below is a list of key information and ideas to take away from your reading supported by Nurse Hopen's own words (Hopen, personal communication, December 1, 2021).

- *"It's important to bring your whole self to your practice."*
- *"I try to take care of the patient and treat their situation, as if the patient is my own relative or loved one."*
- *"I felt very blessed to have really good relationships with the other Nurses. So, to have time to decompress [caring for self] and to talk about what was going on with the other Nurses [Nurse-to-Nurse caring]."*
- The call for *unknowing* is choosing to be open in *heartmindbodysoul* to come to know other in the moment.

## End-of-Chapter Questions, Applications, and Group Activities

**Directions:** Use what you have learned in this chapter to reflect upon and respond to the questions, applications, and group activities below.

### Questions

- In "*Struggling to Walk the Walk*," how did Nurse Hopen come to know what mattered most to the patient?
- What other calls for Nursing are present in this Nursing Situation?

### Applications

- Reflect on a time when a call for unknowing, as a pattern of knowing, was manifested in your own Nursing practice.

### Group Activities

- Nurse Hopen identified Boykin and Schoenhofer's theory (2021), *Nursing as Caring,* as guiding her practice. Identify key components of the theory and Nursing Situation that support this. What other caring theory of Nursing do you see as guiding Nurse Hopen in her practice? Why?
- Informed by her EBP, Nurse Hopen co-created a holistic healing environment in response to what mattered most to persons experiencing gender affirmation surgery. Then think about how the reflective reflexive process is manifested within mutual process and knowingdoing-becoming. How does she co-create a holistic healing environment within which suffering is transcended through and within healing?

8

# "Listen to My Voice"

## Introduction

In this chapter, we present Christopher Demezier, DNP, CNM, who has practiced in intensive care for three years followed by becoming a certified Nurse midwife. He shared the core tenets of his Nursing practice that remain the same within any setting.

> *Effective communication with the healthcare team but also with the patient—a willingness to take a step back and work with the patient and let the patient take the lead. And I think that another tenet that's really big for me is almost like an attention to detail. I think patients and staff and other members of the healthcare team are in tune with people who can pick up on the small details. I think that really does guide my practice well.* (Demezier, personal communication, November 18, 2021)

Nurse Demezier reflected on his thoughts about healing.

> *So, for me, healing is not necessarily achieving "optimum health," right? We can throw medication at everybody; we can throw as much oxygen, throw as many lines and interventions that we can do, but ultimately it's about a person's definition of [wellbecoming]. So, it's not saying like, okay, once your numbers look good then you're healed, so to speak. But if a patient has the satisfaction where they feel that their needs are being met, and they have achieved a goal where they can be an active member of the team, then for me that's a level of healing. And so, like in that regard, someone can be taking a turn towards the end of life. But if that's a goal for them, or something that they've come to accept, then maybe the team may not want that. But if a patient feels like, you know, I don't want to do this anymore, I want to just be comfortable, let me be, then in that regard, not that I'm putting science on hold, but I can honor that person and give them respect that's due. So, at the end of the day, I'm here for them, and if they don't want interventions, then they don't want interventions. So, let's talk about how we can make you comfortable, what can I do. And so, my definition of healing really is talking about the patient's [wellbecoming] as defined by the patient, as opposed to medicine's or Nursing's definition of what healing is in a textbook somewhere.* (Demezier, personal communication, November 18, 2021)

We asked Nurse Demezier, from his perspective, what is an essential element for co-creating a holistic healing environment in practice.

> *I think one is respect. Unfortunately, and maybe this is more like a practical approach, as opposed to an educational or theoretical approach, I feel a lot of Nurses—and maybe this might be an effect of COVID—have lost respect for patients, where, you know, it's either do as I say or I'm not going to help you. There are patients that can be difficult, and I understand that sometimes they may need a more direct approach, but by and large I feel each patient has an individual opportunity to provide care that's directed towards them, and so by walking in with respect you can really provide that for them. You're getting report—you know this patient is very difficult, this patient is white, this patient is withdrawn, or whatever. And unfortunately, that could influence how you approach your patient and that bothers me. So, I keep that in the back of my head. Because you know somebody is difficult, but in the same regard I treat every interaction as an opportunity to demonstrate that I'm here for this patient. I've had several patients that were difficult with other people, but when I had the opportunity to talk with them and sit and really understand their motivations and their feelings and how things were happening, we ended up connecting. I figure out what's important for [the patient], and I use my skills and my knowledge and my experience to optimize that for her/him. I feel that without that, it's just pill pushing, like medication pushing, and that's not what I'm here for. People come to the hospital for Nursing care—not medicine—and in order to do that, I have to be able to respect the person. Respect for person is a central tenet that I feel is important for helping patients to achieve healing.* (Demezier, personal communication, November 18, 2021)

## Objectives

After completing this chapter, readers will:

- Within the Nurse's living experience described in this chapter, identify the patterns of knowing and ingredients of caring.
- Within the HHE Framework, describe the Nurse's *knowingdoingbecoming* as soul whisperer and healer in the context of the Nursing Situation "Listen to My Voice".
- Demonstrate the reflective reflexive process in applying the HHE Framework within the selected Nursing Situation.

## Key Terms and Concepts

**Directions:** Before continuing, we encourage you to take time to refamiliarize yourself with key concepts in Chapter 3, "*Co-Creating a Holistic Healing Environment: The Framework.*"

## Nursing Situation: *"Listen to My Voice"*

Nurse Demezier shared the following Nursing Situation. It is an exemplar of co-creating a holistic healing environment in the moment by focusing on what mattered most to the patient.

> *A 21-year-old first-time mom, and I did a lot of my intrapartum rotation at a military facility, so she was an independent spouse. And unfortunately, her husband was deployed overseas, and so she was by herself. And her family lived eight hours away, so they wouldn't be in time for the birth. She had presented eight centimeters basically ready to go. And this is towards the end of my rotation, and so, for me with gentle instruction from my preceptors, I was able to take control of the labor room. So, things I did to sort of promote that healing environment were: I turned the lights down low and I kicked everybody out of the room who wasn't the immediate Nurse, my preceptor, or the charge Nurse who are there for all deliveries. We got her husband on FaceTime with permission from their commanding officer and he was able to actually be right there next to her and during the whole process. Instead of looking at me, I had the patient look at her husband just so that in that moment as she's pushing, she says, "Listen to my voice." She was able to connect with her husband there in the moment. Thankfully, at her six-week appointment, her husband was able to show up in the office. It was a nice reunion because it was the first time for me meeting him, but it was a reconnection with the patient, and it was nice to sort of come full circle. For me, maintaining the family presence there was really helpful for her in that moment.* (Demezier, personal communication, November 18, 2021)

## Exploring the Emergence of the Holistic Healing Environment Framework

### Through and Within the Reflective Reflexive Process

Let's now explore the emergence of the HHE Framework through and within the reflective reflexive process within his practice and the Nursing Situation *"Listen to My Voice"*. The reflective reflexive process is manifested within mutual process and *knowingdoingbecoming* from which emerges authentic presence, integral presence, and compassionate unity transcending suffering towards healing.

#### *Authentic Presence*

How does Nurse Demezier prepare self for and live authentic presence?

One of Nurse Demezier's central tenets for his practice to co-create a holistic healing environment is respect for person. *"I feel each patient has an individual opportunity to provide care that's directed towards them and so by walking in with respect you can really provide that for them"* (Demezier, personal communication, November 18, 2021). This illuminates Nurse Demezier's awareness of and coming to know self in synchrony and harmony within alternating rhythms guided by Mayeroff's ingredients of caring and Roach's caring attributes to choose *who I bring to practice in this moment.*

Who he chooses to bring to practice in this moment is then manifested as authentic presence when he shared: *"I treat every interaction as an opportunity to demonstrate that I'm here for this patient"* (Demezier, personal communication, November 18, 2021).

### *Integral Presence*

Through *knowingdoingbecoming,* he becomes integrally present through perceiving-experiencing the integrality of himself as Nurse and environment—the wholeness of self and the interconnectedness of self with his patients. In his *knowingdoingbecoming,* integral presence is manifested *within; "when I had the opportunity to talk with them and sit and really understand their motivations and their feelings and how things were happening, we ended up connecting"* (Demezier, personal communication, November 18, 2021).

### *Compassionate Unity*

He then emerges from integral presence to compassionate unity through and within the alternating rhythms of perceiving-experiencing *I feel you, you feel me, and I feel you feeling me* (Hübl, 2021, p. 2)—the interwoven energy field of himself as Nurse, his patient, and her husband, simultaneously the healer and healee, all healing and both being healed. Within the HHE Framework, Nurse Demezier comes to know the patient's call for connection.

His patient was a 21-year-old first-time mom whose husband was in the military. *"Unfortunately, her husband was deployed overseas and so she was by herself. And her family lived eight hours away, so they wouldn't be in time for the birth"* (Demezier, personal communication, November 18, 2021).

Nurse Demezier described taking control of the labor room to co-create a holistic healing environment. *"I turned the lights down low, I kicked everybody out of the room who wasn't the immediate Nurse, my preceptor, or the charge Nurse who are there for all deliveries. We got her husband on FaceTime with permission from their commanding officer, and he was able to actually be right there next to her and during the whole process"* (Demezier, personal communication, November 18, 2021).

The call for Nursing in *any* Nursing Situation is experienced only through compassionate unity, which emerges through mutual process, knowing participation, and *knowingdoingbecoming.* Within compassionate unity, Nurse Demezier co-created a holistic healing environment in an active labor situation with a patient who had no family support. The patient and her husband experienced ease from suffering as Nurse Demezier created an opportunity to connect his patient and her husband via FaceTime.

Nurse Demezier came to know the importance of the energetic connection between the Nurse, his patient, and her husband. Therefore, connecting via FaceTime alone was not sufficient within this Nursing Situation. *"Instead of looking at me, I had the patient look at her husband just so that in that moment as she's pushing, she says, 'Listen to my voice.' She was able to connect with her husband there in the moment"* (Demezier, personal communication, November 18, 2021).

Nurse Demezier, his patient, and her husband are all in a mutual process. Their individual energy fields are integral with the environmental field of the labor room. Within compassionate unity, even though the husband is virtually present, the interconnection between and among them transcended suffering and co-created healing.

Nurse Demezier is soul whisperer and healer.

## Summary

In this chapter, we illuminated Nurse Demezier's practice through the interpretation of the HHE Framework. His *knowingdoingbecoming* has evolved through his years of ICU practice integrating now with his Nurse midwifery practice. Within alternating rhythms guided by Mayeroff's ingredients of caring and Roach's caring attributes, we share in the living experience of who he *chooses to bring to practice in the moment. "People come to the hospital for Nursing care—not medicine—and in order to do that, I have to be able to respect the person. Respect for person is a central tenet that I feel is important for helping patients to achieve healing." Coming to know self and his patients, he lives in integral presence. "When I had the opportunity to talk with them and sit and really understand their motivations and their feelings and how things were happening, we ended up connecting"* (Demezier, personal communication, November 18, 2021).

Through the Nursing Situation *"Listen to My Voice"*, we experience manifestation of Nurse Demezier's authentic presence as he takes control of the labor room emerging to his integral presence as Nurse Demezier, his patient, and her husband (who is virtually present) are in simultaneous mutual process within the interwoven energy field in the labor room. Compassionate unity is radiated through and within Nurse Demezier, his patient, and her husband as he softly tells his patient to focus on her husband *"just so that in that moment as she's pushing she says, 'Listen to my voice.' She was able to connect with her husband there in the moment"* (Demezier, personal communication, November 18, 2021). Within compassionate unity, Nurse Demezier is soul whisperer and healer. This Nursing Situation is an exemplar of the dance of alternating rhythms with intentional knowing participation to co-create an environment through which holistic healing emerges for Nurse and person(s).

## Key Takeaways from This Chapter

Within this chapter, the Nurse's living experience of co-creating a holistic healing environment is revealed through the interpretation of the HHE Framework. Below is a list of key information and ideas to take away from your reading supported by Nurse Demezier's own words (Demezier, personal communication, November 18, 2021).

- Within authentic presence, walk into a person's room with respect. *"I feel each patient has an individual opportunity to provide care that's directed towards them, and so by walking in with respect you can really provide that for them"* (Demezier, personal communication, November 18, 2021).
- Avoid labeling patients as difficult. *"When I had the opportunity to talk with them and sit and really understand their motivations and their feelings and how things were happening, we ended up connecting"* (Demezier, personal communication, November 18, 2021).
- *"I treat every interaction as an opportunity to demonstrate that I'm here for this patient"* (Demezier, personal communication, November 18, 2021).
- When receiving report, do not let judgment statements about the patient influence how you will approach the patient. *"I keep that in the back of my head."*

- *"My definition of healing really is talking about the patient's [wellbecoming] as defined by the patient, as opposed to medicine's or Nursing's definition of what healing is in a textbook somewhere"* (Demezier, personal communication, November 18, 2021).

## End-of-Chapter Questions, Applications, and Group Activities

**Directions:** Use what you have learned in this chapter to reflect upon and respond to the questions, applications, and group activities below.

### Questions

- In "*Listen to My Voice*," how did Nurse Demezier come to know what mattered most to the patient?

### Applications

- Reflect on Nurse Demezier's perspective on what is an essential element for co-creating a holistic healing environment in practice. Then think about how the reflective reflexive process is manifested within mutual process and *knowingdoingbecoming*. How does he co-create a holistic healing environment within which suffering is transcended through and within healing?
    - *"You're getting report, you know this patient is very difficult, this patient is white, this patient is withdrawn or whatever. And unfortunately, that could influence how you approach your patient and that bothers me. So, I keep that in the back of my head.*
    - *When I had the opportunity to talk with them and sit and really understand their motivations and their feelings and how things were happening, we ended up connecting."*
- Reflect on Nurse Demezier's personal definition of healing. How does that resonate with you? How does that resonate with the definition of healing in the HHE Framework?

### Group Activities

- Which caring theory of Nursing do you see as guiding Nurse Demezier in his practice? Why?
- Nurse Demezier *"was able to take control of the labor room"* to *"promote that healing environment."* Identify a situation within your practice where you as the Nurse could take charge and co-create a holistic healing environment.

# UNIT III

# Designing Educational Experiences within the Holistic Healing Environment Framework

## Introduction

In Unit I and throughout the book, we have presented the Holistic Healing Environment (HHE) Framework and its underpinnings. The profound words from the Nurses' living experiences in Unit II were explored within the HHE Framework, which revealed the imperative for healing within and through caring for self to care for another.

In this unit, we now illuminate how the HHE Framework may be manifested within educational experiences. Through discovering the patterns of knowing and ingredients of caring we come to know and appreciate the need for *knowingdoingbecoming* and compassionate unity within praxis and the education of Nurses. Although presented within two individual chapters, the HHE Framework is integral regardless of the educational setting, including curricula within academia (didactic, clinical, simulation experiences) or professional Nurse development within any healthcare system.

The focus of this unit emerges from two questions:

- *Why should we prepare Nurses to co-create a holistic healing environment within practice settings?*
- *How do we prepare Nurses to co-create a holistic healing environment within practice settings: students enrolled in a Nursing program, novice Nurses, and expert Nurses?*

There continues to be an exodus from Nursing as Nurses experience suffering emerging from being devalued and burnout (Morphet et al., 2019; Tinsley & France, 2004; U.S. Bureau of Labor Statistics, 2020). The COVID-19 pandemic further exacerbated this suffering. Without Nurse caring for self in his/her wholeness, there is loss of meaning manifested as a state of suffering commonly understood as *burnout* (Britt, Scholar, & Acton, 2022; Tinsley & France, 2004). Loss of meaning may include loss of self and loss of what it personally means to be a Nurse and to care for self to care for another. This answers the question *Why should we prepare Nurses to co-create a holistic healing environment within practice settings?*

As presented in Chapter 3, the unique focus of Nursing, the call for Nursing, mutual process and knowing participation, *knowingdoingbecoming* as mutual patterning and integration into praxis are the soul of the HHE Framework. As the unique focus of Nursing is healing, *the call for Nursing* is to co-create an environment of holistic healing for the Nurse and other to transcend suffering. The purpose of the framework is to guide the Nurse in concert within caring theories of Nursing in co-creating a holistic healing environment where healing emerges within and through caring. A holistic healing environment, within the HHE Framework, is the dance of alternating rhythms with intentional knowing participation to co-create an environment through which holistic healing emerges for Nurse and person(s).

Within the HHE Framework, it is imperative that Nurse co-creates a holistic healing environment, and we assert that Nurse is soul whisperer and healer. **This ... is ... Nursing!**

9

# The Call to Care for Self to Care for Another

## Introduction

*Newly graduated nurses are entering the work force and finding that they have neither the practice expertise nor the confidence to navigate what has become a highly dynamic and intense clinical environment burdened by escalating levels of patient acuity and nursing workload* (Duchscher, 2008, p. 441).

The words above were printed in 2008, 12 years before the COVID-19 pandemic impacted Nursing education and praxis and the entire healthcare system. Now more than ever, a framework is needed to prepare Nursing students to co-create a holistic healing environment. The Holistic Healing Environment (HHE) Framework presented in this book answers that call.

Nightingale's theory supports that the Nurse (as soul whisperer and healer) must first come to know and care for self in his/her wholeness—*heartmindbodysoul*—to care for another. Within the HHE Framework, Nurse caring for self in his/her wholeness to care for another is foundational in *knowingdoingbecoming* in praxis. In this chapter, we focus on how to prepare the student in Nursing in coming to know and care for self to care for another. "We cannot know caring unless we have learned it/experienced it from within; for ourself/with ourself, before others" (Watson, 2018, p. xvv).

**Objectives**

After completing this chapter, readers will:

- Understand that Nurse caring for self in his/her wholeness to care for another is foundational in *knowingdoingbecoming* in praxis.
- Appreciate how the Nursing student experiences healing within and through the experience of feeling cared for.
- Integrate the HHE Framework within Nursing curricula and courses for caring for self, manifested in healing and wellbecoming.

### Key Terms and Concepts

**Directions:** Before continuing, we encourage you to take time to review the key concepts in Units I and II. Specifically:

- **Self-care**—Focuses on strategies to address our deficits and weaknesses; often grounded in feeling guilty or being upset with ourselves. A focus on strategies provides a piece-by-piece plan trying to balance everything to fix us.
- **Caring for self**—Holistic blueprint for wholeness and self-healing through coming to know self in our wholeness and what matters most to us within our *heartmindbodysoul.*
- **Inner coherence**—the person's *heartmindbodysoul* is in harmony and synchrony.
- **Resilience**—"The *capacity* to *prepare* for, recover from and adapt in the face of stress, adversity, trauma, or tragedy" (HeartMath® Institute, 2021a, para 3, ln 1–2).
- **Trauma**—"The subjective experience of an event, or series of events, that overwhelms an individual's capacity to cope" (HeartMath® Institute, 2021b, p. 1).
- **Ingredients of caring**—Knowing, alternating rhythms, patience, honesty, trust, humility, hope, and courage.
- **Patterns of knowing**—Are manifested as repeating/enduring waves of *knowing/doing/becoming* that are always integral, evolving, and emerging. Currently there are 11 patterns: aesthetic, emancipatory, empirical, ethical, intuitive, narrative, personal, sociopolitical, spiritual, technological, and unknowing.

Having served in higher education and academia for many years, we know what it feels like when anyone suggests a curricular change. This feeling is rarely one of excitement but rather *here we go again* with more committees, policies, updating courses and syllabi, and on and on. But our promise to you is—choosing where and how to integrate the HHE Framework can be exciting. Faculty may choose to integrate the HHE Framework by focusing on one course, a level of courses such as the first year of the program, or the entire curriculum. We will offer many potentialities on the beauty of integrating the HHE Framework.

So, as we have in previous chapters, we begin with a Nursing Situation.

## Nursing Situation: *"I Am So Scared I'm Going to Flunk Out"*

*As typical in many academic programs, the purpose of the midterm assessment is to help students understand where they are headed in their studies and what, if any, changes need to happen to ensure their success. The advisor had been talking with and studying the patterns of freshman Nursing students for several semesters. Anywhere between 30% and 50% of the students were struggling at midterm, but it was not because they couldn't do the work, even though the work was considerably harder than high school. Although faculty were available to them, the advisor came to know that students were anxious, lonely, homesick—all manifested in missing classes and falling grades before midterm. During midterm conferences, there were students who reported they wanted to drop out and go back home. One student said, "I miss my friends back home. I don't have any friends here. I can't sleep." Another student shared, "I have to work, as my parents can't help me. I am so scared I'm going to flunk out—I can't focus." As she started to cry, a student said, "Sometimes I feel like I can't breathe at the beginning of a class because I didn't do the reading and I'm worried the teacher will call on me." These students were experiencing trauma—"the subjective experience of an event, or series of events, that overwhelms an individual's capacity to cope" (HeartMath® Institute, 2021b, p. 1). In response to student anxiety and fears, the advisor and faculty encouraged students to seek counseling available through student health services. However, students would not keep their appointments due to a perceived stigma.*

**Thoughtful Reflection**

Reflect upon the students' words above that portray their living experience. Which ingredient(s) of caring are needed?

A common misperception is that students know how to take care of themselves—when to sleep, eat, manage their time, and ask for help. Or if we give self-care strategies to students, they will use them to "fix" their deficits. Back in Chapter 1, we differentiated between caring for self and self-care. Self-care focuses on strategies to address our deficits and weaknesses—and they're often grounded in feeling guilty or being upset with ourselves. A focus on strategies provides a piece-by-piece plan trying to balance everything to fix us. Self-care strategies are often unrealistic, we just do not have time, or we are too tired to follow the plan.

This Nursing Situation is greater than taking care of self—it is coming to know self through knowing mutual participation while simultaneously experiencing being cared for and caring for self. It is the call to care for self to care for another.

Caring for self holistically starts with coming to know self in our wholeness and what matters most to us within our *heartmindbodysoul*. Caring for self is grounded in healing and loving; appreciating our strengths as well as what needs to be strengthened; and forgiving our stumbles and blunders. So, caring for self is a holistic blueprint for wholeness and self-healing with integrative daily approaches that helps us strengthen our "*capacity* to *prepare* for, recover from and adapt in the face of stress, adversity, trauma, or tragedy" (HeartMath® Institute, 2021a, para 3). In the Nursing Situation above, each student as energyspirit is experiencing trauma.

Now, let's revisit the Nursing Situation above within the HHE Framework. How might this Nursing Situation unfold as healing through and within caring? Within their wholeness, the advisor and faculty emerge from authentic presence to integral presence and compassionate unity and come to know the student as energyspirit experiencing trauma.

Within the underpinnings of the HHE Framework, students, advisors, and faculty are all in mutual process and therefore perceived as an energy field and may be viewed in two ways:

1. Students, advisors, and faculty may be regarded as a group field, a single, indivisible team-as-group field where students, advisors, and faculty are one in mutual process with the environmental field.

2. Everything other than the "team" can be regarded as its environment. (Rogers, 1990, p. 8; France, 1994, p. 198)

When focusing on the students, advisors, and faculty as individuals, the individual energy fields are integral with the environmental field or the educational setting, which includes the team (Rogers, 1990, p. 9; France, 1994, p. 198). Each team member is a unique energy field in mutual process with the environmental field. Students and advisors/faculty are continuously in mutual process with their environmental fields, which encompass the team. Each individual person is an energy field different from and greater than the sum of parts, and the team-as-group field is different from and greater than the sum of parts; thus, the team is a very dynamic field. The team—students, advisors, and faculty—is co-creating a holistic healing environment to transcend suffering. As students/faculty/advisors are integral and in mutual process, when focusing on students, faculty and advisors must also experience being cared for and caring for self to then care for another. As advisors, faculty and students are in mutual process, all simultaneously experience being cared for, caring for self to then care for another. The student experiences *knowingdoingbecoming* as mutual patterning manifests the wholeness and alternating rhythms of healing and is integral to caring for self, authentic presence, integral presence, and compassionate unity.

## Exploring the Integration of the Holistic Healing Environment Framework

The HHE Framework can be integrated at many levels and/or in several stages—by individual faculty within courses, the overall curriculum, and organizational system. We are offering two potentialities: within a course and at the organizational level.

Prior to deciding to make formal curricular changes, individual faculty may initially choose to integrate the HHE Framework within courses at any level. We recommend integrating the framework within the very first Nursing course so students experience the ingredients of caring and being cared for as they come to know how to care for self to then care for another. Within the HHE Framework, experiencing being cared for emerges through the ingredients of caring and helping them come to know self through patterns of knowing such as personal, spiritual, intuitive.

Guided by the HHE Framework, we offer the following potentialities for the student/faculty/advisor as individuals and as team.

- Begin each class or clinical practicum or advising session with a self-awareness practice such as heart-focused breathing (HeartMath®) or a grounding/centering exercise.
    - Based on what is happening in the class, the clinical setting, or the advising session—difficult discussions, exams/quizzes, heart-focused breathing, or an awareness practice—can be added.
    - Develop a consistent practice of caring for self that includes awareness exercises or grounding/centering exercises.

- Schedule time and activities with intention
  - Consider space and time when planning advising sessions, scheduled class time, and/or when developing course offering plans
    - Reflection, meditation, yoga, walks, mindful eating of snacks and meals
    - Schedule meetings/courses with start/end times and an appropriate length of time with adequate breaks
- Teach and integrate reflective practices such as the thoughtful reflections and group activities presented throughout this book

There are outcomes that can be measured to evaluate if faculty, students, and advisors see a difference after initiating the above suggestions. For example, quantitatively, what is the pattern of student grades, attendance, and level of participation? Qualitatively, have students engage in guided self-reflection regarding feelings of stress, if/how/when they may be using heart-focused breathing, or an awareness exercise outside of class.

Following an evaluation of outcomes within courses, faculty may then choose to reevaluate the program's mission/vision/philosophical statements and curricula for integrating the HHE Framework. Again, the HHE Framework does not stand by itself but is philosophically congruent with caring theories of Nursing in the Unitary-Transformative Paradigm. Your mission/vision/philosophy and curricula may already be in harmony to integrate the framework.

While considering potential curricular changes, it is important to include resources to support co-creating healing through and within caring for the team (students/faculty/advisors). For example, given a perceived stigma associated with receiving counseling, the college or university could have board-certified health and wellness Nurse coaches available to students, advisors, and faculty. We are very specific here—Nurse coaches. There are many life coaches, wellness coaches, and caritas coaches out there. The health and wellness Nurse coach (HWNC-BC) is board-certified as a holistic Nurse and as a Nurse coach who guides the student/advisor/faculty in caring for self in his/her wholeness to establish goals for wellbecoming and experiencing *knowingdoingbecoming.*

## Summary

In this chapter, we described why we prepare Nurses to co-create a holistic healing environment and how the HHE Framework can be integrated into Nursing curricula and student experiences. In addition, student activities appear throughout the book. By being immersed within a holistic healing environment, students/advisors/faculty will simultaneously experience being cared for as they come to know self and care for self, strengthening inner coherence and resilience manifested as healing through and within caring. Through caring for self, students then emerge into authentic presence, and as they prepare to care for another, they emerge into integral presence and compassionate unity—Nurse as soul whisperer and healer.

## Key Takeaways from This Chapter

In this chapter, we introduced potentialities on how to integrate the HHE Framework within the academic setting. We invite you to consider the following when co-creating Nursing curricula and redesigning student experiences that support *knowingdoingbecoming*:

- As the HHE Framework is philosophically congruent with caring theories of Nursing in the Unitary-Transformative Paradigm, faculty may see that their mission/vision/philosophy and curricula may already be in harmony to integrate the framework.
- When experiencing an event, or series of events, that overwhelms an individual's capacity to cope, the student is experiencing trauma.
- Given a perceived stigma associated with receiving counseling, the college and/or university can have board-certified health and wellness Nurse coaches available to students, advisors, and faculty.
- As students/faculty/advisors are integral and in mutual process, when focusing on students, faculty and advisors must also experience being cared for and caring for self to then care for another.
- Within the HHE Framework, caring for self is a holistic blueprint for wholeness and self-healing with integrative daily approaches that helps us strengthen our "*capacity* to *prepare* for, recover from and adapt in the face of stress, adversity, trauma, or tragedy" (HeartMath® Institute, 2021a, para 3).
- Integrating the HHE Framework within a course(s) may help students emerge into authentic presence, and as they prepare to care for another, they emerge into integral presence and compassionate unity—Nurse as soul whisperer and healer.

## End-of-Chapter Questions, Applications, and Group Activities

**Directions:** Use what you have learned in this chapter to reflect upon and respond to the questions, applications, and group activities below.

### Questions

- Reflect on your living experiences during Nursing school. When and how would you integrate the HHE Framework?

## Applications

- In caring for self, design a holistic blueprint for your wholeness and self-healing with integrative daily approaches that helps you strengthen your "*capacity* to *prepare* for, recover from and adapt in the face of stress, adversity, trauma, or tragedy" (HeartMath® Institute, 2021a, para 3).

## Group Activities

- As students/faculty/advisors are integral and in a mutual process, when focusing on students, how can faculty and advisors also experience being cared for and caring for self to then care for another?
- Choose a Nursing course from your current curriculum, integrate the HHE Framework into the course description, rewrite one objective, and design one student experience for this objective that supports *knowingdoingbecoming.*

10

# *Knowingdoingbecoming* in Praxis

## Introduction

"It would be logical to assume that unless nurses regularly see to their own physical, psychological, and spiritual/existential [wellbecoming], their ability to provide the highest level of patient care will gradually diminish—a conclusion also acknowledged by Nightingale herself" (Riegel et al., 2021). Nightingale's theory supports that the Nurse as soul whisperer and healer must first come to know and care for self in his/her wholeness—*heartmindbodysoul*—to care for another and team. Within the Holistic Healing Environment (HHE) Framework, Nurse caring for self in his/her wholeness to care for another is foundational in *knowingdoingbecoming* in praxis. In this chapter, we focus on how to help Nurse in coming to know and care for self to care for another and team within the context of pandimensional transition in practice settings.

**Objectives**

After completing this chapter, readers will:

- Understand that Nurse caring for self in his/her wholeness to care for another and team is foundational in *knowingdoingbecoming* in praxis.
- Appreciate how the Nurse experiences healing within and through the experience of feeling cared for.
- Integrate the HHE Framework within Nursing professional development for caring for self and team, manifested in healing and wellbecoming.

**Key Terms and Concepts**

**Directions:** Before continuing, we encourage you to take time to review the key concepts in Units I and II. Specifically:

- **Self-care**—Focuses on strategies to address our deficits and weaknesses; often grounded in feeling guilty or being upset with ourselves. A focus on strategies provides a piece-by-piece plan trying to balance everything to fix us.

- **Caring for self**—Holistic blueprint for wholeness and self-healing through coming to know self in our wholeness and what matters most to us within our *heartmindbodysoul.*
- **Knowing participation**—The intentional mutual patterning within person and environment, which are unitary and inseparable.
- **Unknowing participation**—Lack of awareness and attention to mutual patterning within person and environment, often manifested within a task-oriented practice approach.
- ***Knowingdoingbecoming***—Manifests the wholeness and alternating rhythms of healing *heartmindbodysoul.*
- **Praxis**—The interconnectedness of a discipline's worldview, science, theories, research, education, and practice emerging as "a synthesis of thoughtful reflection, caring, and action within theory and research-driven practice" (Hines & Gaughan, 2014, p. 26); a synchrony of knowing/doing/being (Watson, 2018, p. 21).
- **Inner coherence**—the person's *heartmindbodysoul* is in harmony and synchrony.
- **Resilience**—"The *capacity* to *prepare* for, recover from and adapt in the face of stress, adversity, trauma, or tragedy" (HeartMath® Institute, 2021a, para 3 ln 1–2).
- **Trauma**—"The subjective experience of an event, or series of events, that overwhelms an individual's capacity to cope" (HeartMath® Institute, 2021b, p. 1).
- **Ingredients of caring**—Knowing, alternating rhythms, patience, honesty, trust, humility, hope, and courage.
- **Patterns of knowing**—Are manifested as repeating/enduring waves of *knowing/doing/becoming* that are always integral, evolving, and emerging. Currently there are 11 patterns: aesthetic, emancipatory, empirical, ethical, intuitive, narrative, personal, sociopolitical, spiritual, technological, and unknowing.
- **Transition**—A pandimensional experience manifested as turbulence.
- **Turbulence**—"A dissonant commotion in the flow of human-environmental field patterning characterized by chaotic and unpredictable rhythms" (Smith, 2020c, p. 13). May emerge from excitement, suffering, fear, love, uncertainty.
- **Trauma**—"the subjective experience of an event, or series of events, that overwhelms an individual's capacity to cope" (HeartMath® Institute, 2021b, p. 1).
- **Ease**—"resonant harmony in the flow of human-environmental field patterning characterized by calm and familiar rhythms" (Smith, 2020c, p. 13).
- **Turbulence ease**—"Shifting patterning of turbulence to ease" (Smith, 2020c, p. 18). The Nurse as environmental field integrally present with other can shift the patterning of turbulence to ease.
- **Healing huddle**—A gathering of Nurse and staff with the intention of grounding and centering to knowingly participate as team to move through turbulence to ease for healing.

Many people understand transition as major life events, such as birth, marriage, graduation, and death. Within the Unitary-Transformative Paradigm and the HHE Framework, transition is a pandimensional experience manifested as turbulence moment-to-moment.

The role change from student Nurse to Registered Nurse (RN) is often described as a transition into a new journey of exciting experiences and as a crossing into a reality of the unknown filled with anticipation, and/or anxiety, and/or fear. Transition from student Nurse to RN is not linear. It is pandimensional; therefore, in his/her wholeness, the graduate Nurse experiences transition *heartmindbodysoul.*

It is important to remember, the expert Nurse also experiences transition *heartmindbodysoul.* Commonly occurring transitions include changes in policies, Nurse managers/administration, and staffing and staffing patterns. Changes in staffing and staffing patterns may include the hiring of newly graduate Nurses and working alongside travel Nurses assigned to their unit. Expert Nurses who accept a travel Nurse assignment also experience transition.

Transition has been typically viewed as something to be "managed" in a linear method to prepare the individual Nurse (novice or expert) to "hit the floor running" as soon as possible. Most organizations design programs of transition as a one-size-fits-all approach. Transition is expected to be achieved within a time-specified orientation and/or residency/internship regardless of whether the Nurse is a new graduate, an RN who has transferred units, or a newly hired experienced RN. Regardless of how these linear programs are designed, they are not working. Nurses are leaving the discipline and profession.

Within the HHE Framework, transition is not simply passing from one point to the next, it is pandimensional and experienced simultaneously by Nurse as individual and as team. Transition is manifested as turbulence within the healthcare and practice setting. But turbulence is not always a negative experience. "Both turbulence and ease are necessary for wellbecoming" (Smith, 2020c, p. 16). Smith (2020c, p. 17) reminds us of the

> need to generate some turbulence in our lives to make changes that are necessary for our wellbecoming. This might be accomplished by pushing ourselves out of our "comfort zones", embracing the unfamiliar, re-framing change as necessary for growth and wellbecoming, and becoming more comfortable with the feelings surrounding turbulence without labelling these feelings as "bad."

**Thoughtful Reflection**

As the newly graduated Nurse and the expert Nurse are in continuous mutual process with their environment, how do they seek or offer ease from this turbulence?

## Nursing Situation: *"I'm Good. But I Knew I Wasn't"*

*I've been practicing for 10 years in the acute care setting and within those 10 years, three years as the Nurse manager. The accountability and responsibility of being an RN is unbelievable but even more so as the manager.*

*You have to be ready at any given moment to switch gears, find the answers, jump in. I thought I was doing pretty good within my first year, until one day I wasn't.*

*We had a high-stress event on the unit plus orienting three new graduate Nurses. I called psychiatry, security, and tried to keep Nurses calm as I saw the fear in their faces. I was going 150 miles per hour when I looked up and saw the holistic Nurse from the Integrative Health Department coming towards me. I heard myself say, "I'm good," but I knew I wasn't.*

*The holistic Nurse took me to a private area. After some deep breathing and receiving Reiki, I realized that I haven't been caring for self, and my stress and anxiety were impacting everyone on the unit. I needed help in dealing with the chaos.*

*Although I kept making the excuse of not having time, I began regularly meeting with the holistic Nurse coach. At first, I was hesitant and a little nervous. But, she focused on me, my strengths—not my weaknesses or deficits. I realized that I was coming to know myself again as a person and as a Nurse. As I was rediscovering my love and passion for Nursing, I felt myself healing. My practice began evolving. How could I now help my team to heal, strengthening their resilience?*

*I practiced grounding and centering several times during the day—to help me know who I choose to bring to practice today—before I walked onto the unit, during meetings, and in stressful situations. I discovered that when I'm grounded and centered, I feel more connected—like heart-to-heart connection, feeling joy, and becoming authentically present. I started paying attention to the repeating patterns and rhythms manifested Nurse-to-Nurse, Nurse-to-patient, and other. They, too, were experiencing stress and were showing signs of trauma and suffering from the environment.*

*I requested a holistic Nurse coach be assigned to my unit. I expanded the orientation for the new Nurses to include Nurse coaching sessions but to also be available to coach any Nurses or staff who were interested in learning how to care for self. At the beginning of each shift, I gather the team asking how everyone is doing that morning. I offer an awareness practice to guide them in grounding and centering, becoming authentically present. I am intentionally in-tune with each Nurse as individual energyspirit and the unit as team energyspirit for timely moments of rest, reconnection, healing. As team we are integrally present working in synchrony trusting each person's competence and caring for self, the team, and patient.*

## Exploring the Emergence of the Holistic Healing Environment Framework

### Through and Within the Reflective Reflexive Process

The Nurse manager in the Nursing Situation above *co-created a holistic healing environment by shifting the pattern of turbulence to ease—healing.* Let's now explore the emergence of the HHE Framework through and within the reflective and reflexive process—the *why* and *how* the HHE Framework is essential in Nursing practice through revisiting the underpinnings of the framework.

When focusing on the Nurse manager, new graduate Nurses, experienced Nurses, and staff as individuals, the individual energy fields are integral with the environmental field or the practice setting, which includes the team (Rogers, 1990, p. 9; France, 1994, p. 198). Each team member is a unique energy field in mutual process with the environmental field. Nurse manager, new graduate Nurses, and experienced Nurses/staff are continuously in mutual process with their environmental fields, which encompass the team. Each individual person is an energy field different from and greater than the sum of parts, and the team-as-group field is different from and greater than the sum of parts; thus, the team is a very dynamic field. The team—Nurse manager, new graduate Nurses, experienced Nurses, and staff—is co-creating a holistic healing environment to transcend suffering. As team, Nurse manager/ new graduate Nurses/experienced Nurses and staff are integral and in mutual process. When focusing on the new graduate Nurses (for example), the Nurse manager, experienced Nurses, and staff must also experience being cared for and caring for self to then care for another. The Nurse manager, new graduate Nurses, experienced Nurses, and staff are in mutual process, all simultaneously experience being cared for, caring for self to then care for another. Each person experiences *knowingdoingbecoming* as mutual patterning manifests the wholeness and alternating rhythms of healing and is integral to caring for self, authentic presence, integral presence, and compassionate unity.

*Knowingdoingbecoming* manifests the wholeness and alternating rhythms of healing *heartmind-bodysoul.* As person and environment are in continuous mutual process, transition is inherent within *knowingdoingbecoming* and is manifested as alternating and unpredictable rhythms or turbulence. As Nurse knowingly participates with environment, she/he experiences the turbulence and within integral presence then shifts the pattern to ease—healing. Healing is then experienced by Nurse and other manifested in strengthened inner coherence and resilience to live through transition.

Now, let's revisit the Nursing Situation where the Nurse manager stated, *"I realized ... my stress and anxiety were impacting everyone on the unit. I thought I was good, but I wasn't."* Here she is manifesting *unknowing participation*—not realizing that as she is in mutual process with environment and how she is experiencing alternating rhythms were impacting team. The Nurse manager in essence was increasing the flow of turbulence increasing trauma and suffering.

However, she comes to know that she needed help in dealing with turbulence. Scheduling time with the holistic Nurse coach was her first step in caring for self. With the holistic Nurse coach, *"I realized that I was coming to know myself again as a person and as a Nurse. As I was rediscovering my love and passion for Nursing, I felt myself healing. My practice began evolving."* Through knowing participation, the Nurse manager manifests the wholeness and alternating rhythms of healing *heartmindbodysoul,* which unfolds as she chooses who to bring to practice.

In addition to meeting with the holistic Nurse coach, the Nurse manager continues to explore who she is as person, Nurse, and Nurse manager through reflection and keeping a journal. She wrote:

> *One of the major things I have become aware of is my need to have control. When I feel out of control, I feel vulnerable, anxious, fearful. But I have come to know that I cannot make anything perfect; challenges will arise and it is okay if I do not have all the answers. I am learning how to let things unfold as they are and having the courage to accept uncertainty. I am learning to embrace the unknowns with hope for abundant possibilities.*

Through coming to know self, the Nurse manager in the Nursing Situation above increased her awareness and authentic presence. As she became integrally present, she co-created a holistic healing environment by shifting the pattern of turbulence to ease—healing, thereby strengthening the inner coherence and resilience of team. She came to know that the orientation for new Nurses did not address the turbulence of transition as a pandimensional experience. Therefore, she redesigned the orientation for the Nurses to experience transition in its wholeness. Knowing her expert Nurses and staff may also be experiencing turbulence, she encouraged the team to have sessions with the holistic Nurse coach assigned to the unit and invited them to gather at the beginning of the shift and participate in an awareness practice.

The importance of gathering together as team is to co-create harmony and synchrony. Within the HHE Framework, we use the term *healing huddle* as it is grounded in holism and wholeness for caring for self, caring for team to then care for patient, family, and others. The healing huddle does not replace the team huddle as both are needed. Unlike the team huddles that focus on healthcare team alignment around important daily tasks and actions, the focus of the healing huddle is to bring Nurses and staff together with the intention of grounding and centering to knowingly participate as team to move through turbulence to ease. A healing huddle begins with an awareness practice and can be called at the beginning of the shift, end of the shift, or whenever necessary. While any member of the team can initiate the call, Nurse as soul whisperer and healer is integral to co-creating the healing huddle. Within the healing huddle, healing is then experienced by Nurse and other manifested in strengthened inner coherence and resilience.

Transition is a pandimensional experience manifested as turbulence moment-to-moment with continual changes in the flow of human-environment field patterns. A holistic healing environment supports inner coherence and resilience of individual and team. Within the HHE Framework, transition experiences are redesigned as holistic and pandimensional so individuals and team all simultaneously experience being cared for, caring for self to then care for another.

We offer the following when integrating the HHE Framework to support *knowingdoingbecoming* within healthcare organizations across settings:

- Administrators respect
  - Nurse as co-creator of healing and peace through caring science; helps person to find meaning in the living experience and wellbecoming; soul whisperer, healer.
  - Nursing as a basic and applied science, discipline, art with its own unique, abstract, substantive body of knowledge created from basic and applied research and development and testing of its theories; a learned profession.
  - Nurses as persons who are educated to use Nursing knowledge (science) according to nationally regulated, defined, and monitored standards for the protection and safety of healthcare for society and its members.
  - Nurses have autonomy, responsibility, and accountability for Nursing praxis.
- Nurses co-create transition experiences for individual and team that are holistic and pandimensional.
  - Move away from the notion of a one-size-fits-all linear orientation process to co-creating a culture of a lifelong clinical learning process that is pandimensional and manifested as an expression of caring for the graduate Nurse where the graduate Nurse experiences being cared for.

- ○ Prepares and supports the graduate Nurse to co-create a holistic healing environment throughout her/his career beginning with caring for self and coming to know self in his/her wholeness as energyspirit.

- Nurses and staff as team co-create a holistic healing environment.
    - Assign holistic Nurse coach to unit.
        - Opportunities for holistic Nurse coaching sessions provided by the organization.
        - Formal or informal ways of sharing experiences of Nurse coaching, holistic Nursing, and reflective practice.
        - Opportunities for holistic therapies
            - Massage
            - Energy therapies such as Reiki
    - Co-create a mission/vision/philosophy in synchrony with HHE Framework.
    - Co-create policies and procedures that strengthen Nurse and staff's inner coherence and resilience.
    - Open each shift with a healing huddle.
    - Live caring for self.
    - Experience being cared for and belonging.

## Summary

In this chapter, we described why we prepare Nurses to co-create a holistic healing environment and how the HHE Framework can be integrated into the redesign of Nursing transition experiences. We revisited unitary caring science and HHE Framework underpinning that the individual energy fields are integral with the environmental field or the practice setting, which includes team. As team, Nurse manager/new graduate Nurses/experienced Nurses and staff are integral and in mutual process. Individual and team must experience being cared for and caring for self to then care for another. As Nurse and team are in continuous mutual process, transition is inherent within *knowingdoingbecoming* and is manifested as alternating and unpredictable rhythms or turbulence. As Nurse knowingly participates with team, she/he experiences the flow of turbulence and within integral presence shifts the pattern to ease—healing. Healing is then simultaneously experienced by Nurse and team manifested in strengthened inner coherence and resilience to live through transition.

## Key Takeaways from This Chapter

Within this chapter, the Nurse's living experience of transition manifested as turbulence and coming to know how to co-create a holistic healing environment. Below is a list of key information and ideas to take away from your reading.

- As person and environment are in continuous mutual process, transition is inherent within *knowingdoingbecoming* and is manifested as alternating and unpredictable rhythms or turbulence.
- As Nurse knowingly participates with environment, she/he experiences the flow of turbulence and within integral presence then shifts the pattern to ease—healing.
- Healing is experienced by Nurse and other manifested in strengthened inner coherence and resilience.
- As the Nurse manager increased her awareness and practicing authentic presence, she became integrally present and shifted trauma from turbulence into ease strengthening the inner coherence and resilience of team—co-creating a holistic healing environment.

## End-of-Chapter Questions, Applications, and Group Activities

**Directions:** Use what you have learned in this chapter to reflect upon and respond to the questions, applications, and group activities below.

### Questions

- Reflect on a time when you experienced transition and turbulence. How did you seek ease? Was it through self-care strategies or caring for self in wholeness?

### Applications

- Visualize the Nurse in the Chapter 1 Nursing Situation, *"'I'm Your Nurse. And I'm Here with You,'"* as part of team on the Nurse manager's unit described in this chapter. What connections and/or patterns do you see between the Nursing Situations and the HHE Framework?

### Group Activities

- Have you ever been with a small group of people who were all having a good time and someone joined the group who was in a bad mood? What happened to the group's energy field? Did it shift from positive to negative? Now imagine as Nurse you are experiencing a difficult day. How might the quality of care your patients receive be impacted?
- You're one of the staff Nurses on your unit. There has been much transition and turbulence over the past several weeks. Describe the current environment. How will you co-create a holistic healing environment for team?

# UNIT IV

# Co-Creating a Holistic Healing Environment to Ease Suffering and Restore Humanness and Humanity During Times of War and Pandemic

## Introduction

Up to this point in the book, we have explored together the Nurse in what appears to be everyday practice co-creating a holistic healing environment—in hospitals, private practice, with adults, with children, with communities. So, why is this unit on war and pandemic included? We asked ourselves—What is its purpose? Are these not the worst of the worst conditions to provide nursing care? Is it even conceivable and possible to co-create a holistic healing environment within these conditions? We believe the answer is yes—it is conceivable, it is possible, it is essential! For many Nurses around the world, war and/or pandemic become everyday practice.

The purpose of this unit is to integrate what it means to co-create a holistic healing environment through and within caring under the extreme conditions of war and pandemic to ease suffering for peaceful restoration of our humanness and humanity, in life or death. We acknowledge while as Nurses we do not get to choose those conditions, we are called to co-create healing and peace through and within caring moment to moment. As Nurses, we understand that co-creating a holistic healing environment in today's world in any condition is a moral, social justice imperative. Although war and pandemic have existed for hundreds of years, more so now than ever Nurses are in the position to influence healing and peace. Remember within the Holistic Healing Environment (HHE) Framework, we define Nurse as: *co-creator of healing and peace through caring science; helps person to find meaning in the living experience and wellbecoming; soul whisperer, healer.*

Chapter 11 begins by presenting a brief history of the role of Nurses during war focusing on specific Nurses who impacted our discipline and profession. Later in this chapter, we present first-hand accounts of Nurses, descriptions of their lived experiences, and Nursing Situations that serve as exemplars of co-creating healing environments on the front lines.

In Chapter 12 we compare and contrast the Spanish Flu of 1918–1919 and the COVID-19 global pandemics and describe the Nurse's *knowingdoingbecoming* as soul whisperer and healer during pandemics. Through the use of shared Nursing Situations, we explore how the Nurse as soul whisperer and healer strengthens resilience and moral knowing.

War and pandemics have existed throughout history and sadly will continue to exist within our world's future. The HHE Framework presented in this book describes the unique focus of Nursing as healing through and within caring and provides the structure needed for Nurses to thrive under the extreme conditions of wars and pandemics and ease suffering of persons, families, and communities.

11

# Co-Creating a Holistic Healing Environment in War

> *War (noun)—Hostile contention by means of armed forces, carried on between nations, states, or rulers, or between parties in the same nation or state; the employment of armed forces against a foreign power, or against an opposing party in the state* (Simpson & Weiner, 1988).

## Introduction

Throughout history, Nurses have been active in wartime. Prior to Nightingale's first formal school of Nursing, persons (mainly women) volunteered as "self-made" Nurses to care for wounded and sick soldiers and community members impacted by war. With the advent of formal education and the creation of the American Red Cross Nursing Service and the Army Nurse Corps, Nurses chose to serve their country through their science, knowledge, and skill.

It is beyond the scope of this book to examine all wars within which Nurses have served or to identify all the Nurses who served. Therefore, this chapter addresses wars and/or conflicts of great historical significance in understanding the evolving roles and contributions of Nurses in co-creating a holistic healing environment, including the Crimean War, American Civil War, Spanish American War, World War I and II, and the Vietnam, Iraq, and Afghanistan wars.

This chapter begins with a brief historical overview of self-made Nurses and educated Nurses, all of whom served during war and in war zones. This chapter also portrays how throughout history military Nurses who were either deployed overseas or assigned stateside did not allow gender and racial prejudices to prevent them from using their knowledge, skill, and commitment as healers and soul whispers to care for soldiers and civilians. Even in war, within *knowingdoingbecoming,* Nurses co-create a holistic healing environment and forge a new path for Nurses in the future.

### Objectives

After completing this chapter, readers will:

- Discover the historical impact of Nurses' co-creating a holistic healing environment during war/conflict.
- Describe the application of the Holistic Healing Environment (HHE) Framework during war in selected Nursing Situations.

### Key Terms and Concepts

**Directions:** Before continuing, we encourage you to take time to become familiar with key concepts integral to understanding how to apply the HHE Framework during war.

- **War** (noun)—Hostile contention by means of armed forces, carried on between nations, states, or rulers, or between parties in the same nation or state; the employment of armed forces against a foreign power, or against an opposing party in the state (Simpson & Weiner, 1988).
- **Humanitarian**—A person promoting human welfare and social reform (Merriam-Webster, n.d.-a).
- **Humanitarianism**—Showing concern for the welfare of humanity; being in a situation in which many human lives are in danger of harm or death (Free Dictionary, n.d.).
- **Self-made Nurses**—Persons (primarily women) portrayed as humanitarians easing the suffering of soldiers, protecting their dignity, and preserving their humanity.
- **Caring for self**—Holistic blueprint for wholeness and self-healing through coming to know self in our wholeness and what matters most to us within our *heartmindbodysoul.*
- **Healing**—Nurse as soul whisperer is integrally present and in compassionate unity with other to ease and transcend suffering.

# The Historical Impact of Nurses during War

*"I stand at the altar of those murdered men and while I live I fight their cause"*

(Nightingale, cited in Dunphy, 2020, p. 38)

## Crimean War (October 1853–February 1856)

The Crimean War involving Russia, France, the United Kingdom, and Sardinia was one of the first conflicts in which the military used what was then considered to be modern technologies such as "mass-produced rifles, exploding shells, sea mines and armoured coastal assault vessels with long-range cannons" (Andrews, 2013, para 6). It was also the first war to be extensively documented as forces communicated via telegraph, "civilian journalists sent dispatches from the battlefield" (Andrews, 2020, para 9), and photographers brought the war to life by producing "hundreds of wet-plate images" (Andrews, 2020, para 11). As a result, the horror of the battlefields with wounded men, disease, and illness was relayed to the public and the Crimean War became known for its logistical and tactical failures and mismanagement of medical supplies (Greenspan, 2019; Andrews, 2020).

Two months into the war, Florence Nightingale arrived in Crimea with "38 handpicked Nurses who had no formal training" (Dunphy, 2020, p. 40). She and her Nurses discovered "the soldiers were poorly cared for, medicines and other essentials were in short supply, hygiene was neglected, and infections were rampant" (Fee & Garofalo, 2010, p. 1591). Nightingale described the conditions she and her Nurses encountered upon arrival at the Barrack Hospital in Scutari: the wounded men laid on "unwashed floors crawling with vermin"; "using their boots for pillows, no blankets, wrapped in their greatcoats ... stiff with blood and filth"; "1000 men suffering acute diarrhea and only 20 chamber pots"; "liquid filth floated over the floor an inch deep ... within the filth lay the men's food" (cited in Dunphy, 2020, p. 40). "The death count was the highest of all hospitals in the region" (Fee & Garofalo, 2010, p. 1591).

Nightingale and her Nurses quickly set about co-creating a healing environment by setting up a diet kitchen and establishing the provisions of "cleanliness, order, encouragement to eat, feeding, clean bed linens, clean bodies, and clean wards ... essential to recovery" (cited in Dunphy, 2020, p. 40). Upon Nightingale's insistence, the British prime minister sent a sanitary commission to open the channel through which the water flowed to the hospital, "flushed and cleansed the sewers, lime-washed walls, tore out shelves that harbored rats, and got rid of vermin" (Dunphy, 2020, pp. 40–41). "Miss Nightingale's anticontagionism was sealed as the mortality rates began showing dramatic declines" (cited in Dunphy, 2020, p. 41).

After spending 22 months in the Crimea war zone, Nightingale returned to England August 7, 1856. Building on her education, practice, and wartime validation of her ideas, she started the first formal education/training of Nurses in 1860.

#### *Self-Made Nurses*

"Self-made" Nurses are persons who have no formal education and are portrayed as humanitarians easing the suffering of soldiers, protecting their dignity, and preserving their humanity. As it is beyond the scope of this book to present all self-made Nurses throughout world history, we have chosen to focus on Nurses serving during the American Civil War.

### Civil War (1861–1865)

Despite Nightingale starting the first Nursing education program in England (1860), formal Nursing education had not yet reached the United States at the start of the American Civil War in 1861. When the Civil War erupted, the term *Nurse* described service that was provided, treating *Nurse* and *Nursing* as verbs and not as nouns. Therefore, self-made Nurses (primarily women) were understood to perform tasks/activities for the comfort of the sick guided only by personal and spiritual knowing and intuition as learned from and/or working side-by-side family or ancestors. Their *knowingdoing-becoming* was not informed by science or empirical knowing.

Despite this limitation, women played a significant role serving as caregivers and co-creating a holistic healing environment in the Union and Confederate hospitals and while working close to the battlefields. Two extraordinary women considered first and utmost as humanitarians presented are Harriet Tubman and Clara Barton.

Although her actual birthdate is unknown, Harriet Tubman was born into slavery in 1820 in Dorchester County, Maryland, and escaped to freedom in the North in 1849. Known for her heroism in freeing slaves and the underground railroad (Biography.com Editors, 2021), often left out of history is that Tubman was also a self-made Nurse. She not only cared for those who she rescued on the underground railroad leading them to freedom, Tubman also worked as a self-made Nurse for the Union Army during the Civil War. She cared for soldiers both black and white by using her expert skill with roots and herbs to restore them to health (Bradford, 1886, as cited in Singleton, 2019). She was considered an expert in herbal medicine and was "so well known for her ability to cure men of dysentery that she was asked by Army surgeons to use her nursing skills to support troops at a military base in Florida" (New York State Nurses Association, n.d., para 6).

In 1862, Tubman went to Beaufort, South Carolina, to serve as a Nurse and a teacher for the Gullah people who had been abandoned by their owners. Then in 1865 she traveled to Fort Monroe in Virginia where she accepted an appointment as matron of a hospital to care for sick and wounded Black soldiers (Singleton, 2019).

One year after Tubman was born, Clara Barton was born in Massachusetts, on December 25, 1821. The youngest of four siblings, Barton was educated as a teacher and started teaching at the age of 17. After years of teaching in Oxford, Massachusetts, which had free public education, in 1850 she furthered her own education. After one year of study, she moved to New Jersey. When she discovered New Jersey had no free public schools, in 1852 she decided to open the first free public school in New Jersey. Given the success of her school, the community built a new larger schoolhouse in 1853 and in 1854 hired a man to be the principal. Barton resigned and left teaching (Clara Barton Birthplace Museum, 2017).

Barton moved to Washington, D.C., in 1854 and worked as a desk clerk in the U.S. Patent Office becoming one of "the first women to gain employment in the federal government" (American Red Cross, n.d.-a, para 1). When her position was eliminated in 1856, she returned home to Massachusetts for a few years; however, upon the election of President Abraham Lincoln in 1860, she once again had a position as a copyist in the U.S. Patent Office (MacLean, n.d.). Then in 1861, the Civil War began, and the newly recruited Union troops poured into the city. Within all the chaos, Barton provided clothing, bedding, food, and supplies to the soldiers. Through her persistence, she obtained "passes" from the government and the army to bring supplies directly to the battlefield and field hospitals. As the war was ending, Barton wrote to families who were seeking information on the soldiers reported missing. Again, in her persistence, President Lincoln wrote: "To the Friends of Missing Persons: Miss Clara Barton has kindly offered to search for the missing prisoners of war. Please address her ... giving her the name, regiment, and company of any missing prisoner" (American Red Cross, n.d.-a, p. 3, para 2).

Establishing the Office of Correspondence with Friends of the Missing Men of the United States Army and running it for four years, Barton and her assistants "received and answered over 63,000 letters and identified over 22,000 missing men" (American Red Cross, n.d.-a, p. 3, para 2).

In 1869, Barton was introduced to the International Red Cross and in 1870 actively responded to serve with volunteers during the Franco-Prussian War. "To protect herself with the newly accepted international symbol of the Red Cross ..., she fashioned a cross out of red ribbon she was wearing" (American Red Cross, n.d.a, p. 4, para 2). Barton founded the American Red Cross in 1881 at the age of 59 and led it for the next 23 years. It was during the Spanish American War 1881 that Barton also expanded the direction of the American Red Cross.

> The American Red Cross moved in a new direction near the end of Barton's tenure as head of the organization when we delivered supplies and services to Cuba during the Spanish-American War. Recipients of Red Cross aid included members of the American armed forces, prisoners of war, and Cuban refugees. This was the first time that the American Red Cross provided assistance to American armed forces and civilians during wartime. (American Red Cross, n.d.-a, p. 6 para 3)

**Thoughtful Reflection**

Let's take some time now to review and reflect upon the incredible humanitarian work of Tubman and Barton during a time when there was no formal education and recognition of Nurses. Within this brief presentation above, let us identify the ingredients of caring (knowing, alternating rhythms, patience, honesty, trust, humility, hope, and courage) and their patterns of knowing (empirical, personal, aesthetic, ethical, spiritual, emancipatory, sociopolitical, narrative, intuition, technological, and unknowing).

Can you identify examples of holistic healing within their service?

### *Formal Nursing Education and Impact on War*

Thirteen years after Nightingale started the first modern Nursing school, formal Nursing education began in the United States under the vision and leadership of Louisa Lee Schuyler. Schuyler was not a Nurse. During the Civil War, at the age of 24, she was one of the organizers within the Women's Central Association of Relief (WCAR) in New York City, which worked in conjunction with the U.S. Sanitary Commission. WCAR's mission was to participate in war relief efforts such as "fundraising, registering female nurses for work in military hospitals, and helping to direct returning, discharged soldiers and soldiers' families to local relief agencies for assistance" (Haley, 2013, para 1). In 1881, Schuyler organized a citizen group of women to visit local jails and hospitals. However, in 1872, Schuyler then created the State Charities Aid Association (SCAA) to formalize these citizen groups that "consisted of volunteer members; men and women from all walks of life" (VCU Libraries Social Welfare History Project, n.d., para 1) and continued frequent visits to jails, hospitals, schools, and asylums (Encyclopedia.com, 2019). Under Schuyler's leadership when the SCAA discovered the "deplorable conditions of the poor houses" and the unacceptable conditions within the wards of Bellevue Hospital, the SCAA submitted a report to the State Board of Charities (VCU Libraries Social Welfare

History Project, n.d., para 1) and applied for permission to establish a training school for Nurses to greatly improve these conditions. Concurrently, they formed a committee to start a training school and obtained support from the medical staff at Bellevue Hospital, who sent Dr. W. Gill Wylie, house surgeon, to Europe to visit Nursing schools. Wylie returned home with many ideas and "a letter of advice and support from Nightingale" (Bradley-Sanders, n.d., para 1). Approximately 13 years after Nightingale started the first modern Nursing school, Schuyler and her team successfully opened the Training School for Nurses. It was the first school in the United Stated based on Nightingale's Nursing principles (Bradley-Sanders, n.d.).

**Thoughtful Reflection**

There are different definitions of training, but it generally refers to learning the skills necessary for a given job or activity. What is the difference between training and education? Why was the advent of formal education of Nurses so important, and how might education impact co-creating a holistic healing environment?

## Spanish-American War (April 21, 1898–August 13, 1898)

Military Nursing became a practice role after the Civil War and with the establishment of educational programs/schools of Nursing. At this time, only men could be military Nurses because women were seen as 'out of place' in the military. However, with the onset of the Spanish-American War which resulted in many war casualties, a typhoid epidemic, and the unsuccessful use of untrained infantrymen as medical corpsmen, many more Nurses were needed (Higgins, 1996). In response, "the surgeon general authorized the appointment of Nurses who would serve under contract to the military. The authorization did not specify a required gender, so women applied" (Duquesne University School of Nursing, para 4). "The nurses selected for Army duty during the Spanish-American War were held to high standards including graduation from an approved school of nursing" (Higgins, 1996, p. 472). As a result, the first all-graduate Nursing service to staff military hospitals was established.

Upon their arrival to Camp Thomas in Chickamauga, Georgia, the chief field surgeon Colonel John Van Rensselaer Hoff shared that they "did not know what to do with a contingent of women in the camp" (Goldenberg, 1992, p. 49); however, it did not take him long to wonder what they would have done without them. There were 45,000 soldiers living in deplorable conditions with the triple scourge of typhoid, malaria, and measles. Under the supervision of Nurse Anna Maxwell, 160 Nurses cared for 1,000 sick men with only 67 deaths (Graduate Nurses in the Spanish-American War, n.d., & It happened Here: Anna Maxwell, n.d.). "More soldiers died of disease than combat. ... The role of skilled graduate nurses in the care of the wounded and military was solidified. ... We cannot do without them" (cited in Graduate Nurses in the Spanish-American War, n.d., para 7).

How did the Nurses respond to the conditions in which they were called to practice? To provide care for the soldiers and maintain sanitary conditions, they worked 14-hour shifts with 20-minute lunch breaks and provided/laundered/maintained their own uniforms. They were paid $30/month plus an allowance for railroad fare to their assigned locations, meals, and occasional lodging. Even in 1898 there was a Nursing shortage as there were not enough Nurses to care for the soldiers, leading to the exhaustion and illness of many Nurses themselves. According to records, no Nurses were killed in combat, but 153 died from diseases (Arlington National Cemetery, n.d.).

It is difficult to find the names of Nurses who served during the Spanish-American War except for two—Clara Maass and Jane Delano. Born and raised in New Jersey and graduating from the Newark German Hospital School of Nursing in 1895, Maass volunteered to serve as a contract Nurse with the U.S. Army Medical Department at the outbreak of the war in April 1898. Her first term of service was at army camps in Florida, Georgia, and Cuba. Following the Spanish-American War, Maass continued her service in the Philippines and then back to Cuba.

Throughout her years of service, Maass gained much experience in caring for victims with yellow fever, which drew her to the Yellow Fever Commission. Experimentation was being conducted on yellow fever immunization with the theory that mild cases with prompt hospitalization under controlled conditions would result in recovery and immunity. Based on the hypothesis that yellow fever was spread exclusively by mosquitoes, Maass volunteered to participate in the experimentation allowing herself to be bitten by an infected mosquito. Maass came down with a severe fever and died 10 days later in Havana, Cuba. She was 25 years old. In 1952, the Newark German Hospital, which had meanwhile changed its name to Lutheran Memorial, was renamed the Clara Maass Memorial Hospital (Britannica, 2021).

Jane Delano is another noted Nurse during the Spanish-American War. Delano graduated in 1886 from the Bellevue Training School for Nurses and became the superintendent of Nurses at a Jacksonville, Florida, hospital from 1887 to 1888 practicing during a yellow fever epidemic (Britannica, 2022). Throughout her years in practice, in Arizona she continued caring for patients suffering from yellow fever and developed innovative Nursing procedures such as the use of mosquito netting. From Arizona, she moved to Pennsylvania to serve as superintendent of Nurses at the University of Pennsylvania. Then in 1898 with the onset of the Spanish-American War, Delano joined the American Red Cross and served as its secretary for the enrollment of Nurses (American Red Cross, n.d.-b).

After the Spanish-American War, the Army Nurse Corps (ANC) was created in 1901 to increase the supply of Nurses to serve in war. Knowing that increasing numbers of Nurses alone was not enough, Delano returned to Bellevue Hospital in 1902 to serve as its superintendent of the Nursing school bringing with her "revolutionary ideas for the nursing curriculum" (American Red Cross, n.d.-b, p. 2, para 2). In 1909, she became the chairperson of the new National Committee on Red Cross Nursing Service and superintendent of the ANC (1909–1912). During this time, she focused on the "importance of having a ready supply of nurses in case of military conflict" "to avoid the lack of preparation the country faced to meet nursing demands during the Civil War and the Spanish-American War" (American Red Cross, n.d.-b, p. 3, para 3). "Under her skillful leadership, the American Red Cross Nursing Service became the recognized nursing reserve for the Army, Navy and Public Health Service" (American Red Cross, n.d.-b, p. 3, para 3). Delano had accomplished her mission of preparing a ready supply of Nurses for war.

## World War I (1914–1918)

The ANC had been in existence for 17 years when the United States entered WWI on April 16, 1917. The Corps was not as large as the American Red Cross Nursing Service with only 403 Nurses on active duty and 170 reserve Nurses as compared to the 8,000 Nurses in the Nursing service reserves of the American Red Cross (Army Nurse Corps Association, n.d.). However, within "six months after the U.S. entered WWI nearly 1,100 nurses were serving overseas in nine base hospitals; ... one year later 2,000 Regular Army and 10,186 Reserve Nurses were on active duty serving at 198 stations worldwide; and by the end of the war the ranks of the ANC increased to 21,480 with over 10,000 having served overseas. This was an increase of 3800% from before the war" (Army Nurse Corps Association, n.d., para 7). As in the Civil War and Spanish-American Wars, during WWI, Nurses served stateside as well as on the enemy front lines. The American Red Cross recruited over 22,000 female Nurses to serve in the U.S. Army between 1917 and 1919. More than 1,500 Nurses served in the U.S. Navy during this period, and several hundred worked for the American Red Cross. Initially during WWI, Nurses were not to face danger near the battlefield. However, those plans had to be changed. When medical groups were reorganized into surgical and gas treatment teams to move specialty care closer to the patients, Nurses became the key team members serving at front-line casualty clearing stations or with forward units. "Ultimately, U.S. nurses worked on surgical teams, hospital trains, hospital ships, and in all sorts of hospitals: field hospitals, mobile units, base hospitals, evacuation hospitals, camp hospitals and convalescent hospitals" (Army Nurse Corps Association, n.d., para 10).

Although the American Red Cross recruited 22,000 Nurses between 1917 and 1919, it is important to understand how a Nursing shortage quickly developed during WWI. Several factors significantly contributed: the Nurse qualifications for the army, base hospital design, the formula of Nurses required to care for patients, and the redesign of medical teams to move Nurses to the front lines. In the beginning, Army Nurses were required to be female, single, age 25–35 years, graduates of training schools that offered both theoretical and practical Nursing, and Caucasian.

Base hospitals were designed as 500-bed hospitals providing definitive treatment for patients transported from the battlefield and evacuation hospitals. The formula of Nurses required for war time had stayed unchanged since the American Revolutionary War (1775–1783) at one Nurse for every ten hospital beds or 50 Nurses for 500 beds. However, even with the formula, someone determined that 46 female Nurses were sufficient for staffing despite that Base Hospital #10 received 1,400 patients during its first week of operations with most of them being surgical patients and mustard gas cases. Nurse Emma Elizabeth Weaver, who worked at Base Hospital #20, reported that "the maximum number of patients in the hospital at one time was 2,275 [in a hospital staffed for 500 beds] ... Grand total of patients admitted was 8703" (Army Nurse Corps, n.d., para 12).

Then as the influenza epidemic hit in 1918 coinciding with WWI, the Nursing shortage became even more severe both overseas and stateside. After first estimating that 10,000 Nurses would be sufficient, "by the end of March 1918 the surgeon general asked for 40,000 nurses" (cited in Army Nurse Corps Association, n.d., para 10). Recruiting Nurses to go overseas then impacted the number of Nurses needed stateside as well. In addition to the gross miscalculation of Nurses needed, the U.S.

military's rejection of African Americans or immigrant Nurses to serve overseas despite drafting men from these groups significantly contributed to the Nursing shortage (Jones, n.d.).

In spite of a Nursing shortage, Nurses answered the call to care for soldiers on the frontlines and at home working 12–14-hour shifts. For the first time in history, the Army awarded Nurses with medals and rank in recognition of their service in which their *knowingdoingbecoming* dramatically improved patient mortality and morbidity in war on the frontlines of battle (Army Nurse Corps Association, n.d.). Let us now introduce you to two Nurses whos served with distinction during WWI: Sara Sand Stevenson and Aileen Cole Stewart.

What we know about Sarah Sand Stevenson is from her first-hand account of serving in World War I. Following her death in 1975 at the age of 90, her family found two trunks of carefully preserved Nursing memorabilia and a typed manuscript describing her service during World War I. The book is written in first person directly from the heart and experience of Nurse Sarah Sand Stevenson. Born in Norway in 1884, she immigrated with her parents to the United States in 1892 settling in Emerado, Grand Forks County, North Dakota. She had seven sisters and two brothers. She entered Nursing school at the age of 16, graduating in 1905 with a diploma in Nursing. In 1915, she graduated from the University of North Dakota with a bachelor's degree in Nursing and joined the newly founded North Dakota State Nurses' Association. In 1916, she was appointed director of Nurses at Bismarck Hospital. In 1917, the United States declared war on Germany. In 1918, she voluntarily entered the ANC, signed up for the Emergency Surgical Unit, and completed basic training in Camp Jackson, South Carolina. She then helped organize Base Hospital #60 for overseas service, which was sent to "the advanced sector of the Lorraine at Bazoilles-sur-Meuse, France" (Stevenson, 1976, p. 12).

Stevenson's records show that after several months of intense military training at Camp Jackson, she and her fellow Nurses set sail on September 28, 1918, aboard the *Leviathan,* arriving in France on October 9, 1918. They traveled four days by train, having only bread and water for nourishment; then one day by truck to another camp where she describes being fed a grand meal of hot hash and warm cocoa from the Red Cross canteen service just prior to being checked into their barracks at Bazoilles-sur-Meuse. The Nurses reported to the frontline the next morning. Although Armistice Day was November 11, 1918, Stevenson and comrades were not discharged to leave France until June 10, 1919. Stevenson wrote throughout her notes how Nurses always worked closely together, looking out after each other and caring for each other.

The long days and nights in caring for U.S. soldiers on the frontline started immediately. Stevenson's first assignment was changing the dressings of 100 seriously wounded soldiers. She kept clear records on the dates, the number of wounded soldiers needing dressing changes and the overall condition of the men. She wrote, "Horribly wounded men poured into our camp ... at night by the Red Cross train" (Stevenson, 1976, p. 46). Their orders were to have their patients in their ward ready to send back as they received the newly wounded. Stevenson then writes that during this time seriously wounded German prisoners of war (POW) were also brought to their ward. The Nurses carefully marked off the ward with white sheets where the POWs would remain with the guards. Stevenson shared that they cared for their soldiers first but then provided the same quality of care to the POWs. Towards the end of the war, she wrote in her notes that she could not understand "how any man could be normal and well after such a terrible experience" (Stevenson, 1976, p. 93). On the very last page of her manuscript, she wrote, "In true life, the World War Nurses could never entirely escape from the thoughts of their wounded and dying comrades" (Stevenson, 1976, p. 112).

The same year the United States entered WWI, Aileen Cole Stewart passed her Nursing exams. She was born in Piqua, Ohio, in 1893, a descendant of former slaves, but we do not know very much about her childhood. In 1914, she was accepted to Freedman's Hospital Training School in Washington, D.C., to study Nursing at Howard University Medical School, participating in the three-year program for African American Nurses to earn their diplomas. The Freedman school had the reputation of being a tough program and preparing Nurses for the difficulties of war. Freshmen student Nurses attended class and worked 12-hour shifts and were responsible for 30 patients with the help of a graduate Nurse only in case of emergency. In their second year, student Nurses cared for patients without the graduate Nurse or Nursing assistant. The third year of the program, student Nurses had gained experience for major and minor surgery.

After graduation, Stewart applied for the Army through the American Red Cross (Alexander, n.d.). As presented earlier, although there was a critical Nursing shortage and desperate need for Nurses to serve in WWI, African American Nurses were not assigned to active duty overseas due to segregation.

Stewart's dedication and courage helped her climb the ranks to become one of the first African American women to serve in the Army Nursing Corps. Stewart was also certified by the American Red Cross and served with 17 other African American Nurses during the influenza epidemic of 1918 (Alexander, n.d.).

African American Red Cross Nurses were called into duty when soldiers and workers began to die of the flu. Stewart and a few other Freedmen's Nurses were sent to areas where the railroad workers were dying quickly. The Red Cross sent Stewart to Putney, West Virginia, with another Nurse. Conditions for the railroad workers soon got worse, and Stewart was sent by herself to a small town called Cascade. She worked alone in the mountains until she received a letter from the director of field Nursing at the American Red Cross asking Stewart to serve.

On December 1, 1918, Stewart began her service in the ANC, along with 17 other African American Nurses. Stationed at Camp Sherman, the African American Nurses lived in segregated areas where they cared for African American soldiers and German prisoners of war. Like Stevenson, Stewart also kept notes about her experiences and wrote:

> *The Story of the Negro nurse in World War I is not spectacular. We arrived after the Armistice was signed, which alone was anticlimactic. We had no opportunity for "service above and beyond the call of duty." But each one of us, in the course of our professional relationships, did contribute quietly and with dignity to the idea that justice demands professional equality for all qualified nurses.* (Stewart, 1963, p. 85)

Despite the need for Nurses and the recognized contributions of African American Nurses during WWI, racial segregation and discrimination continued. It was not until after World War II (WWII) that President Harry S. Truman signed Executive Order 9981 requiring the government to integrate the military. Executive Order 9981 stated that "there shall be equality of treatment and opportunity for all persons in the armed forces without regard to race, color, religion, or national origin" (National Women's History Museum, 2019, para 7).

## World War II (1939–1945)

WWII is recognized as "the largest and most violent armed conflict in history" (U.S. Army Center of Military History, 2003, para 1). More than 59,000 American Nurses served in the Army Nurse Corps (ANC) "under fire in field hospitals and evacuation hospitals, on hospital trains and hospital ships, and as flight nurses on medical transport planes" (U.S. Army Center of Military History, 2003, para 1).

The Nurses' *knowingdoingbecoming* significantly contributed to "the extremely low post-injury mortality rate among American military forces in every theater of the war. Overall, fewer than 4 percent of the American soldiers who received medical care in the field or underwent evacuation died from wounds or disease" (U.S. Army Center of Military History, 2003, para 5). The essential requirement of having the integral presence of Nurses during wartime to co-create a holistic healing environment is evident in these survival statistics.

During WWII, it is reported that 27,000 American military personnel were held as POWs in the Pacific. Among those 27,000 were 77 military Nurses, members of the Army Nurse and Navy Nurse Corps, held captive in the Philippines from 1942 to 1945 (National WWII Museum, 2021).

Upon the first attacks in the Philippines on December 8, 1941, the Nurses shifted from regular pre-war duty to trauma Nursing. "The Army Nurses worked around the clock ... in the jungles of Bataan with 18 open-air wards containing 300–400 patients each, wounded and increasingly sick and weak troops" (National WWII Museum, 2021, para 2). With the fall of Bataan and Corregidor, the Nurses were taken as POWs—the largest group of American women to be captured and imprisoned by an enemy. They became known as the "Angels of Bataan and Corregidor" (National WWII Museum, 2021, para 2).

# Nursing Situation: *The Miracle of Compassionate Unity*

After being taken prisoner in the Philippines, "the Nurses were separated from their male counterparts and held with civilian POWs in the Santo Tomas and Los Banos Internment Camps" (National WWII Museum, 2021, para 1). These internment camps were overcrowded and critically undersupplied, creating the most unsanitary conditions.

How did the Nurses co-create a holistic healing environment under these challenging conditions? The Nurses assisted in establishing Santa Catalina Hospital on the grounds of the Santo Tomas Internment Camp. Even with minimal supplies and severe conditions, they provided lifesaving care to the civilian POWs by mitigating epidemics and caring for patients with injuries, starvation, and disease. These Nurses fought for their survival and the survival of others as they waited to be liberated. The American Forces successfully liberated the POWs in 1945, three years after being taken captive. Miraculously, all 77 Nurses survived.

How did the Nurses survive? "The ANC leadership is largely credited with their group's survival. Chief Nurse Captain Maude C. Davison was 57 years old at capture with decades of service experience, including WWI" (National WWII Museum, 2021, para 5). Second in command was the 47-year-old Lt. Josie Nesbit with 22 years of military service (National WWII Museum, 2021, para 5). Through the commanders' integral presence, the Nurses experienced compassionate unity and Nurse-to-Nurse caring within which a purpose and reason to survive emerged. Davison and Nesbit established a regular daily schedule of Nursing duty organized in four-hour shifts. This schedule provided the Nurses time for rest to care for self so they could then care for others (National WWII Museum, 2021). Nesbit lived Nurse-to-Nurse caring. "When a nurse was too weak to work, Nesbit often substituted herself for that nurse's shift. ... She'd find bits of cloth for underwear and tiny pieces of meat for extra protein" (Burrows, 2020, para 18). Davison and Nesbit co-created a holistic healing environment of Nurse-to-Nurse caring within which the miracle of compassionate unity was manifested.

### *Conversations with Nurses Who Served in the Military*

Up to this point, we have relied on historical reports and personal, written narratives to tell the story of the contributions of Nurses co-creating healing environments. In this next section, we will share excerpts of conversations with Nurses who served in conflicts or wars including Vietnam, Iraq, and Afghanistan. In addition, Nurses were asked to share a Nursing Situation that exemplified co-creating a holistic healing environment during war.

## Vietnam War (1954–1975)

The Vietnam War is defined as a protracted conflict between North Vietnam and South Vietnam with its ally United States. From August 4, 1964 to January 27, 1973, the total number of persons who served in all U.S. Armed Forces was 8,744,000 (U.S. Department of Veterans Affairs, 2011).

Our first interview was with Dr. Marilyn "Dee" Ray, RN, PhD, CTN-A, FSfAA, FAAN, FESPCH (hon), FNAP, HSGAHN, Hon. LL. D, a retired colonel in the U.S. Air Force (M. Ray, personal communication, November 3, 2021). She joined the U.S. Air Force in 1967 and served as a flight Nurse during the Vietnam conflict. She shared a little about her experience; however, she was very clear that she would not share anything regarding the political nature of the conflict. She began by saying, *"I got the opportunity to be with the Vietnam War wounded"* (M. Ray, personal communication, November 3, 2021). As a flight Nurse, Ray's unit traveled across the Pacific, with the large C-141 aircraft carrying up to 150 patients from Vietnam to offload in Alaska or California. The missions could be 18 hours long.

During the Vietnam war, flight Nurses held high responsibility and accountability. As there were no physicians on board the aircraft, the flight Nurse was assigned as the medical crew director and co-commanded the flight with the pilot. *"In those days you were called a Co-Commander of the aircraft as you could co-command with the pilot—if you had to change direction and change altitude; land a plane before it was authorized ... if you had a patient turn bad. You could radio ahead to Hawaii to the military hospital there, talk to the emergency room doctor"* (M. Ray, personal communication, November 3, 2021). The flight Nurse medical crew director and the pilot also made the decision if the plane had to "ditch into the sea or crash into land" (M. Ray, personal communication, November 3, 2021).

The Flight Nurse designated as the medical crew director would receive the patient manifest from the Nurse in Vietnam called "Nurse of the day." The Nurse of the day preparing the manifest assessed each patient and determined who was able to fly based on diagnosis, mental state, as well as tolerance of the 18-hour flight. Ray stated, *"That was a big job to assess all those patients and make a decision on who was able to fly"* (M. Ray, personal communication, November 3, 2021). The Flight Nurse as medical crew director then used the manifest to determine how to position patients in the aircraft. Ray pointed out how the Flight Nurse had to know the aircraft they would be flying to determine patient positioning. *"Infected patients would be placed in the rear. Burn patients would not be placed on the same aircraft as infections and they would be placed in the rear. The neuro patients were positioned in the center of the aircraft where the aircraft is the most stable one direction on ascent to prevent blood from pooling in their head and then the opposition direction on descent"* (M. Ray, personal communication, November 3, 2021). Patients with abdominal wounds, orthopedic diagnoses, eye wounds—all were placed in their specified area of the aircraft. If they were transporting patients with addiction problems and who could potentially have drugs, guards were added to the crew. No one on the aircraft carried weapons except for the guards.

The crew assigned to the flight could include additional flight Nurses, medics, guards, and flight technicians. Ray pointed out how she did not meet her crew beforehand, and she had to rely on them to be trustworthy, knowledgeable, and skilled. Even within these circumstances, she co-created a holistic healing environment. For example, she would have a talk with the whole crew and make sure that everybody was on the same page. *"So, I used to give them my report in the morning before we took off. It was always in a special place usually where we gave medication or filled our meds for distribution—where it was quiet. And I used to tell them that I wanted a quiet aircraft. ... Because those planes were long and noisy anyway ... no windows—this was hard on wounded people who were coming home and of course they were all scared. ... Trying to have your whole staff be respectful and quiet. We tried to be as positive as possible, trying to keep the aircraft and personnel quiet. Speaking softly and quietly to the patients, trying to calm them. Because if one patient goes berserk that's the end. I had people who said to me I had the quietest aircraft—what a big blessing for me and very beautiful feedback"* (M. Ray, personal communication, November 3, 2021). Dr. Ray shared the following Nursing Situation that exemplifies co-creating a holistic healing environment during a flight on a C-141 aircraft bringing wounded soldiers from Vietnam back to American soil.

## Nursing Situation: *"Let Me Smell the Earth"*

*On a mission from Vietnam to Alaska with wounded soldiers, one of my patients was a young man who had lost his eyes. Once we were airborne, he said to me "Nurse, when we get to Alaska will you take me out and let me smell the earth?" And I'll never forget it because he wanted to smell as he couldn't see. He was ambulatory so he could walk. It was cold—I dressed him in his coats and when we got to our landing point in Alaska, I took him down the ramp to the tarmac. He knelt down kissing the cold tarmac praying and thanking God. And I am with him, and I'll never forget it because it was so profound for me to have a young guy who was maybe 20 years old with no eyes and his whole life ahead of him to really learn how to live without his eyesight. It was a very profound experience for me to take care of him and provide for his wish to be able to smell the earth."*

## Iraq War (2003–2007; 2009–2011)

The United States initiated war on Iraq on March 19, 2003, and declared an end to the war on December 15, 2011 (History.com Editors, 2003). Due to the length of the war, and the involvement of two or more states, the Iraq War is described as a protected international armed conflict under international humanitarian law (Fleck, 1995).

Dr. Marcia Potter, USAF, RN, DNP, FNP-BC, FNAP, FESPCH, a retired colonel in the U.S. Air Force, began her military career as a turbo prop mechanic enlisting upon graduation from high school. After four years in the military, she graduated with her associate degree in Nursing and then took advantage of an educational opportunity to become a family Nurse practitioner (FNP) from associate degree to master's degree.

*"When I graduated with my FNP degree I got a job in primary care private practice, and I thought it was going to be just absolutely the perfect thing. And then September 11 happened. And I thought sometimes you can have everything and then you can realize that your dreams were a little too small for what you're intended to do"* (M. Potter, personal communication, November 11, 2021). She shared how she was watching a newscast where the commanding general for Walter Reed was being interviewed stating that he needed Nurses to take care of the wounded in body, mind, and spirit. *"I turned to my husband, I said, 'I think that's me.' So, we had a lot of discussion and prayer and I applied to go back into the air force"* (M. Potter, personal communication, November 11, 2021).

Potter went into the reserves as a clinical Nurse for six months and then active duty as an FNP. She was deployed three times: in Germany, Iraq, and Afghanistan. In all her deployments, she ran the primary care clinics, but in Iraq she was deployed to care specifically for women's health needs as the only other healthcare provider was a surgeon. *"My really specific job was to take care of women's health needs, and there were 30,000 women deployed to Iraq spread all over that country"* (M. Potter, personal communication, November 11, 2021).

Although her clinic had standardized hours, she and her team quickly recognized that women could not always get to them when they needed to. *"We were simply on call when their command would notify us that they were incoming. We'd meet them at the air terminal, they get off a helicopter, we take care of them, and then we get them back on the next helicopter back to their mission, if possible"* (M. Potter, personal communication, November 11, 2021).

*"So, lots and lots of moving parts ... in Iraq. My team and I would go to the emergency room, and we would pick out the patients who really didn't need emergency care to leave spaces available for when emergencies really came in"* (M. Potter, personal communication, November 11, 2021). Potter explained how there was never open space, as her unit typically *"got 650 mass trauma victims a month, on average, and most of those people need between six and nine major surgeries just to be able to restore at least partial function and save their lives"* (M. Potter, personal communication, November 11, 2021).

*"This is Iraq, this is pretty much the height of the insurgencies, the car bombings, the suicide bombings. And there was a bombing ... at a mosque ... during the hours when the women and children could worship—176 women and children. So, there were 100 casualties from the bombing, and we got 37 of them in nine minutes. You don't have the right to say no, no more beds, no more space, no more hands—you can't—all you can do is say yes and here's how we do it. We move, we reposition, we reallocate, we do everything we can. So, you just absolutely make room"* (M. Potter, personal communication, November 11, 2021). Potter shared the following Nursing Situation in which she co-created a holistic healing environment for a child injured in Iraq that also provided healing for others.

## Nursing Situation: *Goodnight Moon*

> *I volunteered over at the hospital in my off hours; I was sometimes waiting for patients and sometimes just because in a war zone there's not a lot to fill up your empty time. And so, I worked in the Iraqi*

> *ward. Now the coalition forces including the American soldiers had plenty of people to take care of them so it's not like I was turning my back on them, but the local nationals were strapped for Nurses to take care of them. So, there was a little girl from that mosque bombing, and her mother had been killed and she was two years old and, of course, preverbal and now traumatized—two-year-olds don't know their name, they don't know who their mom or dad is, right? She lost a leg at the knee from the blast, so she's in our ward and we didn't have enough cribs so she was in a playpen and I went over there every night; she is kind of a handful for the Nurses. She's two. She's got a wound vac on. Her whole world is just gone; nobody she knows is around her. And so, every night I would go over there, and I would feed her dinner, and then I give her a bath and then I would rock her for a while. And I would read to her. Now, I know she doesn't understand English ..., but the last book we read every night was Goodnight Moon, so then we will blow kisses, then "goodnight moon, goodnight stars, goodnight Mommy, goodnight Daddy." And then I would tuck her into her playpen. So, in that ward is probably six or seven other young Iraqi victims and only a couple of them had a parent with them. But one of the fathers wouldn't talk to anybody. He hated us, just absolutely hated us, and he didn't like us touching his son and he was just a handful, and the interpreters really had a time with him. So, one night when I'm taking care of this little girl, I hear this noise behind me, and I turn around and it's this Iraqi father and he's got tears in his eyes and he's blowing kisses to this little girl. He looks at me and he said, "You love her," and I said yes. And he said why? And I said because she needs us. So, the next day I come in. On his son's bed there are all these other little children and he's talking to them and he's reading to them and he's polite to the Nurses, and he is finally wanting to trust that we are going to take care of them. Just a small thing to take care of this little two-year-old, but it changes the world for a lot of different people. You have to be able to say I'm going to risk—that man could have killed us. We had people arrested in our wards weekly who were insurgents, who we didn't know at the time that we were taking care of them, but they wanted to kill us, and he could have but instead he began to trust us and it started with that question: Why do you love her? Why do you love anyone? So that is my one of my favorite stories from one of the most horrible places that you can imagine. It makes me tear up.* (M. Potter, personal communication, November 11, 2021)

## Afghanistan War (2001–2021)

The Afghanistan War was triggered by the 9/11 attack on the United States in 2001. The war began on February 29, 2020, and withdrawal of U.S. troops was completed August 30, 2021 (NDTV, 2021). LTC Paul Steven Phipps, CRNA, DNP, is a lieutenant colonel in the U.S. Army and a certified Registered Nurse anesthetist (CRNA) who served in Afghanistan 2020–2021 with Special Forces. *"The typical role of being in Afghanistan is usually being part of an FST, which is a forward surgical team structure that dramatically morphed to being much more mobile"* (P. Phipps, personal communication, November 4, 2021). He explained that by breaking the structural part of the individual components of the FST, the ring of action can be moved to the actual front line to take care of supporting missions.

> *That's what I did in Afghanistan. We were part of what's called the DCRT (damage control resuscitation team) so basically, it's you, a surgeon, and an RN who will serve as a scrub. ... You*

> *are literally on the front lines with command and control literally with the forces when they're taking injuries and hits so you're sustaining them. You're trying your best to stop the bleeding and get them out of the theater as soon as you possibly can and sometimes at that point, you know, you decide when the mission is over. Even if the targets are not actually acquired when you have extinguished your capability of providing that required golden hour, that medical support for that patient mission is suddenly at an end. So that's a realm of Nursing that I never thought that I would actually be in—going to a commander and saying your guy's hit, your mission's over with. And you know, you really, in that role, have to be an advocate saying, I can no longer support any more combat casualties. This mission is at its end, and we have to leave. That was something I think you learn in time—that you really have to be a compassionate advocate at that point for your patients, for your soldiers.* (P. Phipps, personal communication, November 4, 2021)

Phipps talked about how in the military and, especially in a war zone, *"you value the contribution that every team member brings to the situation because you understand that you have a sliver of the situation. And it's everyone coming together contributing that is going to make this situation—this mission—successful. You must see the person behind the role—not as the role"* (P. Phipps, personal communication, November 4, 2021).

He went on to say how he tries to see *"the divine in everything you do and every person that you interact with and every patient that you take. Maybe it's a very philosophical way of looking at it, but I find that, especially after coming back from Afghanistan where life had appeared to have very little value, that that's something that propels me when I'm taking care of my patients. Sometimes you might have a difficult patient or that difficult staff member, but you try to see that divine in that person and it makes it a lot easier to be cooperative and to understand and try to work to accomplish a common goal"* (P. Phipps, personal communication, November 4, 2021). Phipps shared the following Nursing Situation in which he co-created a holistic healing environment with a young solider while under fire.

## Nursing Situation: *"Hold My Hand"*

> *We were on a DCRT mission with special forces. We were in this mud hut in the middle of the night in Afghanistan and you're thinking why in the name of Christ are you even here? I'm thinking that this is such a waste of life. All this stuff is running through your mind.*
>
> *There was this young soldier, a medic. He probably was, I guess, maybe 23 or 24. His name was Daniel. Daniel got hit. It was obvious there was nothing that we could do for him, nothing—he was bleeding out so badly. There comes a point in anesthesia that you clearly can't give anesthesia because it literally will knock out their blood pressure and the idea was to try to keep them perfusing as the surgeon's trying to pack them with trying to do everything. And I was going to give the kid some ketamine so that at least there's some analgesia because I'm feeling terrible for this young man.*
>
> *He grabs my hand, and he says, "I'm not gonna make it." And I'm like, you know, what do you say at that point? You know all the humanity is stripped away from you, you're a human being dealing with another human being who's probably not going to make it home—you know that. You think of all the future that this young man had ahead of him.*

*And he just said to me, "Hold my hand." I held his hand as he passed away. That's all I could do. And that's exactly what you do because behind the soldier is a human being—someone's kid.*

*That kind of weighs on you and it's a sad situation and those faces are still with you at night. And they're always there, you know, they're always there.* (P. Phipps, personal communication, November 4, 2021)

## Applying Holistic Healing Environment Framework during War

We've been reading about courageous Nurses who co-created a holistic healing environment through and within caring during war time and studied specific Nursing Situations that served as exemplars. Now let's explore how to apply the HHE Framework during war from another perspective. The authors visited Arlington Cemetery and spent time at the Vietnam Women's Memorial in Washington, D.C. The Women's Memorial commemorates the 265,000 women who served in the Vietnam War, many of whom were Nurses. The bronze structure depicts three women attending to a wounded soldier, reflecting the unity required during the conflict (Washington, D.C., n.d.).

## Nursing Situation: *Compassionate Unity*

Although this memorial was designed to represent all women who served in various roles during the Vietnam War, we experienced the women depicted in the memorial as Nurses. Within the HHE Framework, the unique focus of Nursing is healing through and within caring. The structure depicts Nurse-to-Nurse caring as well as Nurse-to-soldier caring and exemplifies co-creating a holistic healing environment grounded in unitary caring science. Personal photos of the memorial and an interpretation and perception of the meaning of this memorial within the HHE Framework are shared.

The memorial can be experienced as (1) three Nurses as a team or as (2) one Nurse co-creating a holistic healing environment. (See Figure 11.1).

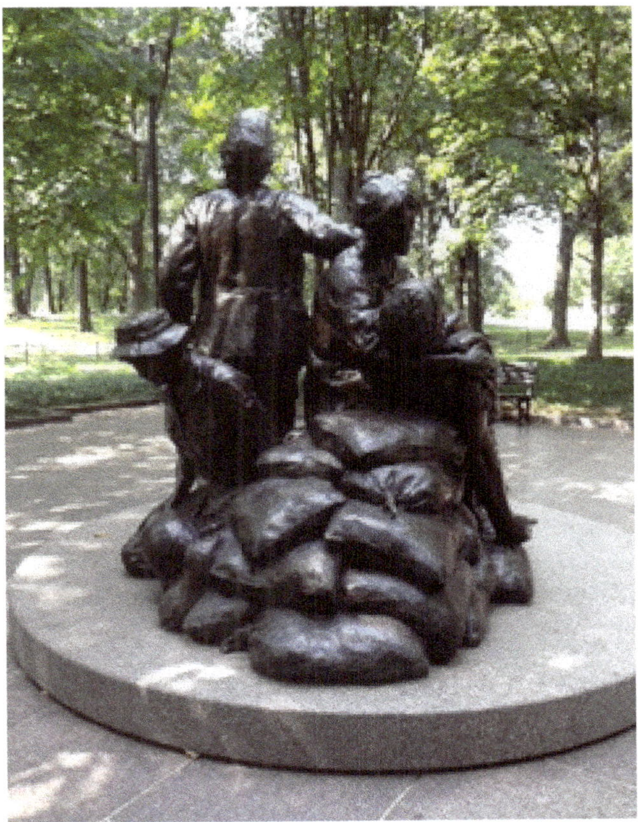

**FIGURE 11.1** Three Nurses as Team Co-Creating a Holistic Healing Environment in Nursing Practice. Statue is Copyright © 1993 by Vietnam Women's Memorial Foundation. Photo by Nancey E.M. France.

At first glance, what do you see in this first picture? We see Nurse-to-Nurse caring as well as Nurse-to-soldier caring. These critical concepts were also manifested by the Nurses who shared their living experiences and Nursing Situations with us earlier in this chapter.

- *Nurse holding soldier*—She cradles the soldier in her lap and focuses on his face.
- *Nurse looking at the sky watching for incoming*—She has her hand on the one Nurse's shoulder and with her body shelters the other Nurse kneeling by sandbags.
- *Nurse kneeling by sandbags*—Given time to rest, caring for self as she holds the soldier's helmet.

Within the underpinning of the HHE Framework, these three Nurses as a team are perceived as an energy field and may be viewed in two ways:

1. [The team] may be regarded as a group field, a single, indivisible team-as-group field where [Nurses] and patients are one in mutual process with the environmental field.
2. Everything other than the "team" can be regarded as its environment. (Rogers, 1990, p. 8; France, 1994, p. 198)

When focusing on the Nurses and patients as individuals, the individual energy fields are integral with the environmental field or the war zone, which includes the team (Rogers, 1990, p. 9; France, 1994, p. 198). Each team member is a unique energy field in mutual process with the environmental field. Nurses and persons/patients/soldiers are continuously in mutual process with their environmental fields, which encompass the team. Each individual Nurse/person is an energy field different from the sum of parts, and the team-as-group field is different from the sum of parts; thus, the team is a very dynamic field. The team is co-creating a holistic healing environment to transcend suffering. Rogers stated,

> Regardless of the group identified, the group field is irreducible and indivisible to itself and integral with its own environment field. ... The principles of homeodynamics postulate the nature of group field change just as they postulate the nature of individual field change. (Rogers, 1990, p. 8; France, 1994, p. 198–199)

### *Applying the Holistic Healing Environment Framework within the Nursing Situation*

Now, let's experience the meaning of the memorial through the Nurse as soul whisperer and healer co-creating a holistic healing environment.

- *Nurse holding soldier*—As she is clutching her cap to apply pressure to a wound, compassionate unity emerges from integral presence revealing Nurse as soul whisperer and healer to transcend suffering (see Figure 11.2).

In Figure 11.3, the Nurse is integrally present and in compassionate unity with her two Nurses manifested by how she positions herself. She simultaneously places her hand in support on the shoulder

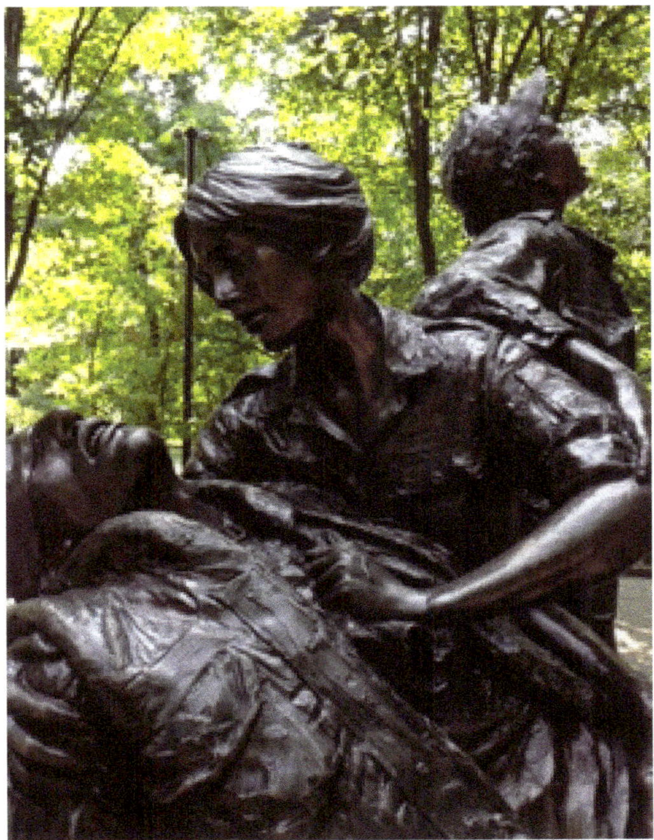

**FIGURE 11.2** The Nurse as Soul Whisperer and Healer. Statue is Copyright © 1993 by Vietnam Women's Memorial Foundation. Photo by Nancey E.M. France.

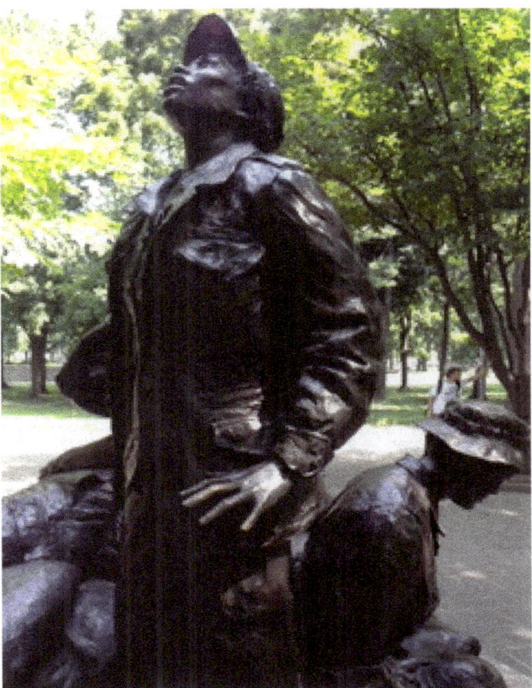

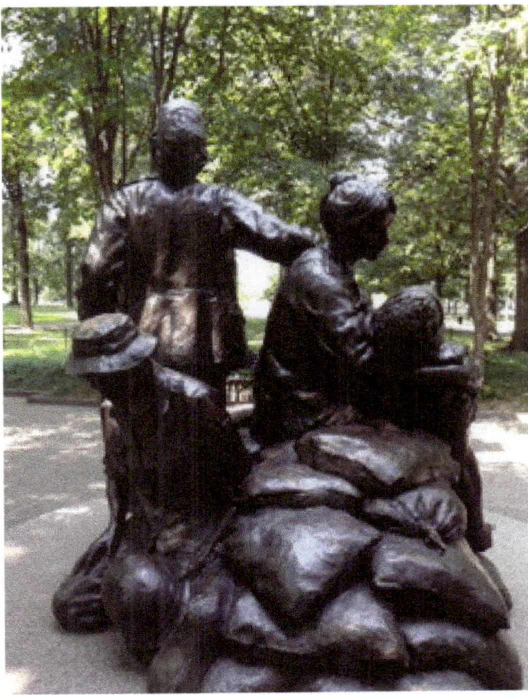

**FIGURE 11.3** Nurse Looking at the Sky, on the Lookout for Incoming. Statue is Copyright © 1993 by Vietnam Women's Memorial Foundation. Photo by Nancey E.M. France.

of the Nurse who is holding the wounded soldier, and she provides shelter so the other Nurse may briefly rest.

In Figure 11.4, the Nurse kneeling by sandbags accepts the given time to rest. She is caring for self, yet she is integrally present so as to be immediately available when needed to answer calls for Nursing. She holds the wounded soldier's helmet in compassionate unity.

## Summary

This chapter began with a selected historical overview of Nurses (self-made/formally educated) who served during war and in war zones. Even in war, within

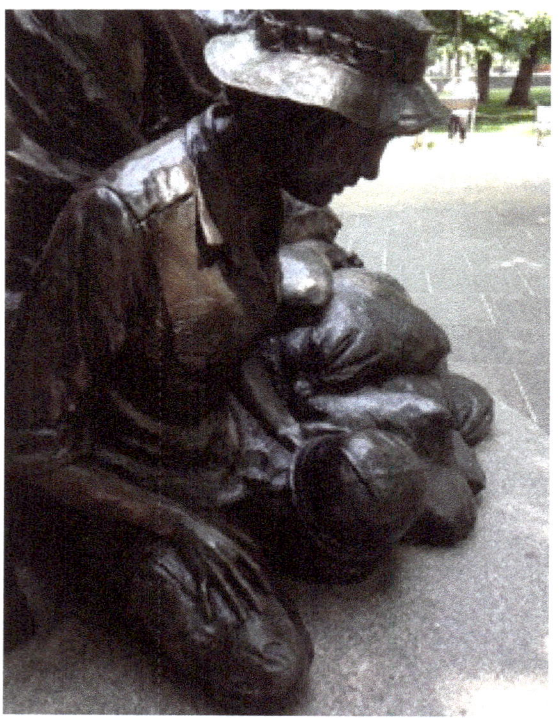

**FIGURE 11.4** Nurse Caring for Self so She Can Then Care for Other. Statue is Copyright © 1993 by Vietnam Women's Memorial Foundation. Photo by Nancey E.M. France.

*knowingdoingbecoming,* Nurses co-created a holistic healing environment through and within caring, forging a new path for Nurses. Within the HHE Framework, even during war, the Nurse as soul whisperer and healer eases suffering for peaceful restoration of our humanness and humanity, in life or death.

## Key Takeaways from This Chapter

The historical impact of Nurses' co-creating a holistic healing environment during war/conflict is revealed through historical reports, personal written narratives, and conversations with Nurses who served during war time. Below is a list of key information and ideas to take away from your reading.

- Prior to Nightingale establishing formal education for Nurses, Nurses were "self-made" and portrayed as humanitarians easing the suffering of soldiers, protecting their dignity, and preserving their humanity.
- Even in war, within *knowingdoingbecoming,* Nurses co-created a holistic healing environment through and within caring, forging a new path for Nurses.
- Within the HHE Framework,
  - the unique focus of Nursing in war is healing through and within caring.
  - even during war, the Nurse as soul whisperer and healer eases suffering for peaceful restoration of our humanness and humanity, in life or death.

## End-of-Chapter Questions, Applications, and Group Activities

**Directions:** Use what you have learned in this chapter to reflect upon and respond to the questions, applications, and group activities below.

### Questions

1. Throughout the chapter, Nurses' *knowingdoingbecoming* is revealed through the patterns of knowing and ingredients of caring in co-creating a holistic healing environment during war.

a. Reflect upon which patterns of knowing and ingredients of caring that were prominent and/or necessary and why.
b. Describe one example of when the Nurse's sociopolitical knowing influenced co-creating a holistic healing environment.

## Applications

1. Within the HHE Framework, identify how the Nurses who have been in war became authentically present, emerged from authentic presence to integral presence and from integral presence to compassionate unity. Look back through the chapter and select two specific Nurses.
2. Hundreds of Nurses who served in the U.S. Armed Services are laid to rest in Arlington National Cemetery, Section 21, also referred to as the Nurses Section. Visit the following sites and describe the two distinct memorials in the Nurses Section:

**Arlington National Cemetery: A Resting Place for Nurses Who Served in the U.S. Armed Services**

**WEB LINK:** https://bit.ly/3PANpS5

**Spanish-American War Nurses Memorial**

**WEB LINK:** https://bit.ly/3MN4YfF

3. In caring for self,
   a. Reflect upon and journal how you experienced this chapter.
   b. Describe how you interpret the meaning of the Vietnam Women's Memorial.

## Group Activities

- In the chapter, you were presented with several Nursing Situations. Choose one and apply the HHE Framework.
  - Ask yourself: *How did the Nurse come to know the call for Nursing to co-create a holistic healing environment during war time*?
  - Which caring theory of Nursing do you see as guiding the Nurse in the Nursing Situation you chose. Why?

12

# Co-Creating a Holistic Healing Environment in Pandemic

*Pandemic (noun)—"an outbreak of a disease that occurs over a wide geographic area (such as multiple countries or continents) and typically affects a significant proportion of the population"* (Merriam-Webster, n.d.-*b*)

## Introduction

In this chapter, we present the stark reality of Nursing during pandemics and the impact of Nursing on persons, families, communities, and society. When there is no cure or when a vaccine may not be enough, within the Holistic Healing Environment (HHE) Framework, the Nurse as soul whisperer and healer eases suffering for peaceful restoration of our humanness and humanity, in life or death. Within the HHE Framework, the Nurse as soul whisperer and healer strengthens resilience and moral knowing in caring for self to care for other.

We begin by providing background information of two of the deadliest pandemics in history: the Spanish Flu 1918–1919 and COVID-19. While separated by 100 years, these two different, yet very similar, viruses brought the world to its knees, burying its citizens. Without medical cures, Nurses with their *knowingdoingbecoming* struggled and fought to ease suffering of persons, families, and communities on the frontlines of a pandemic just as they did during wartime. Parallels between the two pandemics are presented showing the historical, political, and socioeconomic perspectives and the impact upon Nurses and those they care for. The chapter closes featuring three Nurses as soul whisperer and healer and their stories of resilience and moral knowing.

**Objectives**

After completing this chapter, readers will:

- Compare and contrast the Spanish Flu 1918-1919 and COVID-19 global pandemics.
- Describe the Nurse's *knowingdoingbecoming* as soul whisperer and healer during pandemics.
- Identify how the Nurse as soul whisperer and healer strengthens resilience and moral knowing.

### Key Terms and Concepts

**Directions:** Before continuing, we encourage you to take time to become familiar with key concepts integral to understanding how to apply the Holistic Healing Environment (HHE) Framework during war.

- **Pandemic**—"An outbreak of a disease that occurs over a wide geographic area (such as multiple countries or continents) and typically affects a significant proportion of the population" (Merriam-Webster, n.d.-b)
- **Spanish Flu**—A global flu pandemic that started as a localized outbreak in a U.S. Army camp in Kansas and spread within days to New York City and then worldwide (Centers for Disease Control and Prevention, 2019)
- **COVID-19**—A global flu pandemic in which the first hospitalizations occurred in Wuhan, China (Senior, 2022), and quickly spread worldwide. It is the first flu pandemic in which effective vaccines were developed.
- **Resilience**—"The *capacity* to *prepare* for, recover from and adapt in the face of stress, adversity, trauma, or tragedy" (HeartMath® Institute, 2021a, para 3, ln 1–2).
- **Moral knowing**—A pattern of knowing concerned with the development of a moral code in Nursing and determining what is morally correct.
- **Caring for self**—Holistic blueprint for wholeness and self-healing through coming to know self in our wholeness and what matters most to us within our *heartmindbodysoul.*
- **Healing**—Nurse as soul whisperer is integrally present and in compassionate unity with other to ease and transcend suffering.

## The Impact of Nurses during the Spanish Flu and COVID-19 Pandemics

A pandemic is understood as "an outbreak of a disease that occurs over a wide geographic area (such as multiple countries or continents) and typically affects a significant proportion of the population" (Merriam-Webster, n.d.-b). Two of the most devastating global pandemics in history are the Spanish Flu of 1918–1919 and COVID-19. There are several parallels between the two pandemics, including that they began as localized outbreaks that spread quickly; they were initially downplayed by authorities; masks and social distancing were deployed as exposure mitigation strategies; a series of devastating waves and/or surges occurred; a significant number of people were infected and died worldwide; and Nurses and other healthcare professionals were called upon to work tirelessly throughout the pandemic, often at great personal risk (Senior, 2022).

The Spanish Flu and COVID-19 both started as a localized outbreak that then spread at what appeared to be lightning speed. The Spanish Flu did not start in Spain but rather in a U.S. Army camp in Kansas, spreading within days to New York City and then worldwide (Centers for Disease Control and Prevention, 2019). For COVID-19, "timelines of first infections, community transmission, and spread remain widely debated"; however, "first hospitalizations occurred in Wuhan, China" in early December 2019 ... and most agree the virus arrived in Western nations (United States, Italy)" in early January 2020 (Senior, 2022, para 4). By mid-March 2020, fear of viral transmission and rising death rates affected daily living activities around the world. In addition, the day-to-day work expectations of Nurses and other frontline providers were dramatically altered as hospitals and clinics filled with persons who were sick and/or dying.

During both pandemics, authorities around the world were reluctant to disclose the spread of the viruses as well as the anticipated morbidity and mortality outcomes of infection (Senior, 2022). For example, following World War I, there were sociopolitical pressures to suppress news about the Spanish Flu. "One hundred years later, ... most experts believe testing, preparation of the healthcare system, and other considerations were slow to develop until declaration of a national emergency on March 13" (Senior, 2022, para 6).

As there was no vaccine with which to prevent the Spanish flu, nonpharmacological exposure mitigation interventions were implemented, including masks and social distancing along with interventions "such as isolation, quarantine, good personal hygiene, use of disinfectants, and limitations of public gatherings, which were applied unevenly" (Centers for Disease Control and Prevention, 2019, para 2). During COVID-19, the same exposure mitigation strategies were used with varying levels of application affecting the viral spread both before and after effective vaccines became available.

During the 20th century (Spanish Flu), people were divided in two camps regarding wearing masks: those who perceived wearing masks as an effective strategy to slow the spread of disease and those who perceived wearing a mask as an "impairment of their civil liberties ... and an impediment against smoking" (Senior, 2022, para 7). In the 21st century (COVID-19), people also debated the merits of wearing masks with concern for personal and community safety against protection of civil liberties and political affiliation (Senior, 2022).

**Thoughtful Reflection**

Let's take time to reflect on similarities of public response to exposure mitigation strategies during the Spanish Flu and COVID-19. As Nurses, what have we learned that will help us prepare for the next pandemic?

Upon examining the number of cases and deaths from the Spanish Flu, the first wave is described as "relatively mild" (Senior, 2022). But as troops moved around the world, the second wave hit late summer/early fall of 1918 impacting "North, South, and Central America, moving throughout Europe, then Asia and Africa" (Senior, 2022, para 11). The second wave was the deadliest and an estimated 35 million people died—"about 70 percent of the pandemic's total" (Senior, 2022, para 11). There were subsequent waves of the Spanish flu in 1919 and 1920. These waves were "not as severe as the second wave, but more devastating than the initial outbreak ... before the virus lessened in severity, beginning the status we now know as seasonal flu" (Senior, 2022, para 12).

### *Vaccine Development*

The Spanish Flu pandemic changed everything—it increased our understanding of the potential severity and rapid worldwide transmission of flu viruses and our awareness of the need for proactive prevention strategies. However, it was nearly three decades after the Spanish Flu pandemic that the first seasonal flu vaccine was approved for civilian use in the United States (Childs, 2021). Almost two decades after approval, the surgeon general recommended an annual flu vaccine for individuals with chronic illness, anyone 65 years and older, and pregnant women. In 2008, the CDC recommended "children 5 to 18 years old be vaccinated against the flu each year" (Childs, 2021, para 6). "Because new strains of influenza appear frequently, the seasonal flu vaccine usually changes each year" (College of Physicians of Philadelphia, 2018, para 5).

The speed at which vaccines were developed in response to the COVID-19 pandemic was unprecedented. In December 2020, approximately 12 months after the first infection of COVID-19 in the United States, the Food and Drug Administration (FDA) and the Centers for Disease Control and Prevention (CDC) approved the first vaccine for emergency use for individuals 16 years and older (U.S. Food & Drug Administration, 2021a). In May 2021, a vaccine was approved for ages 12–15, and on October 29, 2021, the FDA and CDC announced the approval of a vaccine for ages 5–11 years old (U.S. Food & Drug Administration, 2021b). In total, three vaccines from three different pharmaceutical companies were developed and then approved by the FDA and the CDC. The vaccines were available to persons living in the United States at no cost.

Despite the availability of effective vaccines, the spread of COVID-19 continued to occur in surges versus waves around the world with viral mutation playing an important role (Maragakis, 2021). In September 2021, the Delta variant brought the second deadly surge of COVID-19 (Bollinger, Ray, & Maragakis, 2022). In November 2021, the Omicron variant was identified (Bollinger & Ray, 2021). At the time this chapter was written, COVID-19 surges were continuing around the globe.

As with the Spanish Flu, Nurses answered the call to care for persons, families, and communities during COVID-19. Prior to the development of the vaccine and throughout 2021, hospitals were flooded with intensive care units full and no beds available anywhere in the institution. Nurses worked endlessly with limited resources coping with suffering and death on a daily basis. Hospital visiting policies were rapidly adjusted to protect patients and health care workers. Many hospitals instituted "no visitors allowed" policies. As a result, Nurses were not only trying to save patients from this virus but also co-creating ways to help patients communicate with their loved ones. Nurse Debra Packard stated, "It was heart-wrenching to see a wife have to say good-bye to her husband over video" (Spader, 2021). In addition to acute care, Nurses were needed to oversee and administer vaccine programs in their communities. As with the Spanish Flu pandemic, there was a Nursing shortage, which placed an even greater burden on Nurses in all areas of practice.

The COVID-19 pandemic was on news broadcasts globally, nationally, and locally many times a day for over two years. Increasing infection and death rates, vaccination debates and uncertainty, nonpharmaceutical mitigation strategies such as masking, social distancing, isolation from loved ones, quarantine if sick or testing positive, good personal hygiene, use of disinfectants, and limitations of public gatherings took their toll on the sociopolitical climate and the healthcare system. Reports of Nurses exiting their current positions and even the profession due to feeling a loss of support and weakening resiliency also became a major part of the daily news. The workforce shortages were at a critical level for all patients—not just those with COVID-19 (Alltucker, 2021, 3A).

### *Impact on Nurses*

And yet, there were Nurses who tried to find "the upside of a challenging time" (Spader, 2021). Emergency department Nurse Shannen Kane stated, *"We all have a shared understanding that this is a very difficult time and of what we're all going through. We know we're there for each other and ... trying to make work a bit easier across all of the units"* (Spader, 2021). Kane shared that their support of one another and their shared experience strengthened their bond as a team, which "is going to stay with us, leave a lasting impact on Nursing and how healthcare works, and shape our Nursing careers forever" (Spader, 2021).

**Thoughtful Reflection**

Why is it important for the Nurse as soul whisperer and healer to understand the historical, political, and socioeconomic perspectives of a pandemic?

We now invite you to study three Nursing Situations that present Nurses as soul whisperer and healer. As you read the Nursing Situations, reflect on their stories of resilience and moral knowing and identify applications of the HHE Framework.

## Nursing Situation: Aileen Cole Stewart: *"I'll Go"*

> *The sheets were bloody, they always were. No matter how many times they were changed, the blood kept oozing, dripping from their ears and noses. The young nurse would wipe it, but it continued to trickle over their cheeks where mahogany spots had appeared. She knew in days the spots would disappear, blending into their faces that would turn dark blue from lack of oxygen. In this pre-antibiotic era, death was imminent. All she could do was keep wiping, trying to make them comfortable, until the fluid in their lungs suffocated them. (cited in Cogan & Smilios, 2020, para 3)*

The year the Nursing Situation was written is 1918. With only a year of Nursing experience, Aileen Cole Stewart found strength and courage as she faced WWI and the Spanish Flu pandemic. This pandemic, now in its second wave, deadlier and roaring across the world, was ravaging her country (Cogan & Smilios, 2020). Serving with the American Red Cross, Stewart and two other Nurses were sent to Charleston, West Virginia, to a high school building that had been commandeered to accommodate overflow flu cases from local hospitals. *"When we arrived at the high school ... we were told ... all the patients in the units had died"* (Stewart, 1963, p. 86).

Stewart and the other two Nurses waited for their new assignment from Major Maxwell, the medical director. He showed them a map dotted with white-headed pins indicating critical areas "where a Red Cross Nurse was needed not only for the Nursing care she could give, but also to help a community organize to take care of itself" (Stewart, 1963, p. 86). There were also red-headed pins on the map indicating where Red Cross Nurses were already assigned. Although some of the larger communities had several red pins, most of the areas had only one indicating "there was one Nurse working alone" (Stewart, 1963, p. 86). Pointing at the central and western parts of the state, the commander told them how the miners "are dying like flies. We've got to save their lives ... keep the transports moving. If we keep the transports moving, we can keep our boys crossing over. ... the outcome of the war depends on them and on you Red Cross Nurses" (Stewart, 1963, p. 86). Stewart and one Nurse were assigned to an area that took 24 hours by train to reach. Upon arrival, they walked up the hill behind the station carrying their suitcases shivering with cold. A Miss Blaikney met them and provided breakfast as they made plans for the day. *"Then we all went to work, even though [we] had been traveling more than 24 hours"* (Stewart, 1963, p. 87).

Stewart was assigned to go with the Red Cross physician, Dr. Watts, to visit 20 houses, some of which had several family members who were bedridden. While taking temperatures and providing medications such as aspirin and a cough mixture, they *"talked hospitalization to those with the highest temperatures"* (Stewart, 1963, p. 87). The hours slipped away, and they found themselves eating supper tired and looking forward to going to bed. However, shortly after going to bed, Miss Blaikney knocked on their door bringing them bad news. A Nurse was needed in Cascade, a mining town, and one of them would have to travel that very night. Stewart heard herself say, "I'll go" (Stewart, 1963, p. 87). Dressing warmly "in two sweaters, a coat, a wool scarf and tough shoes" (Stewart, 1963, p. 87), she was on her way to Cascade in a very cold, old Ford. She observed the miners lived in shacks built on stilts because the only road oozed mud during rainy weather. Other than the cook at the commissary, Stewart was the only woman who lodged at the boarding house. She met Joe, the superintendent, who proved to be her right hand. She writes,

> *He knew the men and their problems and could tell me which ones needed help. He made visits with me in the shacks to introduce me to the men, and back up in the hills where the men with families lived. We checked every shack. I made out a written report for Dr. Watts. With three counties to cover, his visits were brief, but he could be counted on when he was needed. By November 11, a field hospital for six of the sickest miners was a reality, set up in a room over the commissary. The only casualty so far in Cascade was an infant.* (Stewart, 1963, p. 87)

## Nursing Situation: Sarah Sand Stevenson: *"The Nurses Remained"*

In the previous chapter, we read about Nurse Sarah Sand Stevenson co-creating a healing environment during war. However, she also experienced caring for others during the Spanish Flu pandemic. In 1918, she voluntarily entered the Army Nurse Corps to serve in WWI, but just a few days after setting sail to France, Stevenson became very ill. "All went well until one day during our lifeboat drill, I became desperately ill. I had the flu." She writes how the Nurses helped each other even though they were sick with the flu, too.

> *As days passed my condition became more serious until one day my true and tried friend came in to see me. She had worked all day and night. This time she picked up my hand and noting its purple color and my serious condition with hemorrhage from my nose, ears, and throat, she said very sadly, "Have you any message to send back to your people? I fear you are about to die. I will deliver it if I return alive."* (Stevenson, 1976, p. 34)

The living conditions on board were deplorable. Stevenson described how the portholes of the ship were allowed open only during the day, which made the night "ghostlike" and the air "was filled with every foul-smelling odor" (Stevenson, 1976, p. 36). During the two-week voyage to France, resources (including water) were limited, and the Nurses were unable to launder bed linens or change their clothes. As they were nearing their destination in France, Stevenson reported all the water on the ship was unexplainably turned off. Dehydrated and becoming even weaker, the Nurses could not walk to the dining room. One of the Nurses found an officer who brought a tray of milk and one piece of sponge cake for each sick Nurse. *"This was a godsend and she [the Nurse] has my everlasting gratitude for this kindness"* (Stevenson, 1976, p. 37).

When they reached port, they were boarded onto a small French boat for transportation to their next location. Stevenson writes, *"There were 20 sick Nurses in this boat; seven were on stretchers. ... we were escorted to the lower decks. Here we stepped around stretchers, literally climbing over the sick and the dying, as the gangway seemed obstructed with them everywhere"* (Stevenson, 1976, p. 37). As they sat on the planks, Nurses on stretchers were placed around their feet. Stevenson noticed one of the Nurses smothering from the blood filling her throat and mouth. "I crept over to her and mopped out her mouth with the corner of her army blanket; we were not so particular at this point of our journey" (Stevenson, 1976, p. 37).

When they reached the next camp of this excursion, Stephenson reports that the American captain "scrutinized each face as we entered" exclaiming, "You all look terrible! What have you got?" (Stevenson, 1976, p. 37). Each Nurse "took the first bed she could stagger to," violently shivering as the corpsmen "helped the captain to pile blankets on us. We had no Nurses as they were rushed beyond endurance with the dying patients who were still on the Leviathan" (Stevenson, 1976, p. 38).

Later that same night, the captain and the corpsmen returned with a cup of hot cocoa for each of the Nurses as well as medicine. *"I think it was laudanum"* (Stevenson, 1976, p. 38). Stevenson reported two Nurses were carried out of the barracks that night and died the next morning. Three days later, the chief Nurse came in notifying "all sick Nurses desiring to go to the Front to be ready to drive out" (Stevenson, 1976, p. 38). After attending the final gas-mask drill, they picked up their helmets, wrote their names across the straps, and went back to their barracks. They were all still weak from the flu.

The next morning there was no conversation in the barracks as the Nurses prepared their belongings. They fell in line standing in the muddy road as they waited to be taken to the truck that would take them to the front. As she stood in line, Stevenson wrote that she let her eyes wander and observed the burial squad carrying the corpses of those who died of the Spanish flu.

"There were fully 2,000 influenza cases on board during the voyage. The Nurses remained until the last sick man was taken off" (cited in Stevenson, 1976, p. 35). Although her experience began with WWI, it is also the backstory of how Nurses and others on their way overseas to France suffered from the Spanish flu. Against this backdrop, the Nurses provided Nurse-to-person and Nurse-to-Nurse care.

**Thoughtful Reflection**

How can the metaphor of "war" help us understand experiences co-creating a holistic healing environment under the extreme conditions of a pandemic?

*Conversation with a Nurse*

Up to this point, we have drawn from historical reports and personal written narratives to describe Nurses co-creating a holistic healing environment during the Spanish Flu pandemic. The next Nursing Situation reflects the experience of a military Nurse co-creating a holistic healing environment while deployed in Afghanistan as the COVID-19 pandemic was developing.

## Nursing Situation: LTC. Paul S. Phipps, CRNA, DNP: *"Come Up with Something"*

LTC. Paul Steven Phipps, CRNA, DNP, is a lieutenant colonel in the U.S. Army and a certified Registered Nurse anesthetist (CRNA) who served in Afghanistan in 2020–2021 with Special Forces. In an interview, he relived the months when COVID-19 hit Afghanistan, forcing a lockdown for several months, and shared the following Nursing Situation.

> *When we were in Afghanistan and COVID was hitting in the States, we knew it was actually hitting in Afghanistan because people were just dying. And they just died as there was minimal care available for those individuals. And suddenly you know that the States were actually getting cut off from us, and we were losing mail connection. We still had that direct military link, but that line was being infringed upon—that resource line in the sense that COVID was actually hitting military establishments, facilities, military bases, military ships, and we were finding out about that. And literally the commander came to us, and we were locked down, which is his right—his capability of locking us down on a FOB, which is a forward operating base in Afghanistan, and telling us we need to come up with a plan off the cuff, something that we can sustain soldiers who come down with COVID. We literally sat down. It was myself, the chief Nurse, the trauma surgeon, the chief of surgery, and we literally sat down in the barracks and within about 48 hours we're coming up with an environment where we could support taking care of soldiers who were coming down with COVID. We didn't have the resources to even create masks. We have digital printers, so we were digitally printing plastic masks and using coffee ground filters. It was pretty astounding. But you know I think there's something that's an intrinsic element in Nurses, is that we can come together, and we can create an environment where we cooperate, work together, and be able to take care of these patients—be able to take care of patients based on what their needs are—and I think that's a*

> *dynamic attribute for experienced Nurses. You can be in an environment, and you can come together, you can have that synergy, and you create an environment where you can take care of those patients.*
>
> *Our FOB was an air force base, which was a huge facility, so it literally became almost like a fortress. It was completely locked down, no one could go in and off the base for several months, and we were locked over there for three or four months. We were constantly going to the CDC guidelines, reaching out to the military trying to create the best attributes that we possibly could. And one of the Nurses literally was reaching back to information from Florence Nightingale during the Crimean War about the sanitary conditions and separating patients. That was the foundation of what we had. It wasn't all the glorious technology that we have. It was doing the best you could—try and create something that could take care of soldiers and patients in a very austere environment* (Phipps, personal communication, November 4, 2021).

At the end of our conversation, Phipps shared with us that no soldiers in his unit were lost to COVID-19 during his time in Afghanistan.

## Applying the Holistic Healing Environment Framework during a Pandemic

We've been reading about courageous Nurses who co-created a holistic healing environment through and within caring during a pandemic and studied specific Nursing Situations that served as exemplars. Now, let's explore how to apply the HHE Framework during a pandemic by taking a deeper look at the Nursing Situation ***"Come up with something."***

In the Nursing Situation ***"Come up with something,"*** Phipps describes co-creating a holistic healing environment while in a locked-down military unit in Afghanistan during the COVID-19 pandemic. They had no "glorious technology," no outside help, and they had to rely on their basic Nursing knowledge. By coming together, they co-created an environment to take care of their unit.

Within the HHE Framework, the unique focus of Nursing is healing through and within caring. By getting back to basic Nursing principles described by Nightingale, Phipps and his team co-created a holistic healing environment under the extreme conditions caused by COVID-19. As you recall from Chapter 11, within the HHE Framework, the unit as a team is perceived as an energy field. In the Nursing Situation ***"Come up with something,"*** the team includes Nurses and all other unit members. Through the Nurses' *knowingdoingbecoming* and integral presence, the team, perceived as a group energy field, is in mutual process manifested as compassionate unity within which suffering is eased and healing is experienced.

## Summary

This chapter presents the stark reality of disease and its impact on persons, families, communities, and society. When there is no cure or when a vaccine may not be enough, within the HHE Framework the Nurse as soul whisperer and healer eases suffering for peaceful restoration of our humanness and humanity, in life or death. The Nurse as soul whisperer and healer strengthens resilience and moral knowing in caring for self to care for other.

## Key Takeaways from This Chapter

In this chapter, we presented the stark reality of Nursing during pandemics and the impact of Nursing on persons, families, communities, and society when there is no cure or when a vaccine may not be enough. Within the HHE Framework, the Nurse as soul whisperer and healer eases suffering for peaceful restoration of our humanness and humanity, in life or death, and strengthens resilience and moral knowing in caring for self to care for other. Below is a list of key information and ideas to take away from your reading.

- There are several parallels between two of the most devastating global pandemics in history: the Spanish Flu 1918–1919 and COVID-19.
- Nurses answered the call to care for persons, families, and communities during the Spanish Flu and COVID-19, working endlessly with limited resources and coping with suffering and death on a daily basis.
- Within the three Nursing Situations, Nurse as soul whisperer and healer co-created a holistic healing environment during a pandemic manifesting resilience and moral knowing.

## End-of-Chapter Questions, Applications, and Group Activities

**Directions:** Use what you have learned in this chapter to reflect upon and respond to the questions, applications, and group activities below.

### Questions

1. Throughout the chapter, Nurses' *knowingdoingbecoming* is revealed through the patterns of knowing and ingredients of caring in co-creating a holistic healing environment during pandemic.
    a. Select one of the Nursing Situations and reflect upon which patterns of knowing and ingredients of caring you perceive to be most prominent and why.
    b. Describe one example of when the Nurse's sociopolitical knowing influenced co-creating a holistic healing environment.

## Applications

1. Select two specific Nurses from the chapter whose described experiences resonate with you. Within the HHE Framework, identify how the selected Nurses became authentically present and emerged from authentic presence to integral presence and from integral presence to compassionate unity.
2. Compare and contrast the *knowingdoingbecoming* revealed in the Nursing Situations described by Stevenson and Phipps.
3. In caring for self,
   a. Reflect upon and journal how you experienced this chapter.
   b. Identify examples of how the Nurses cared for self and how they cared for each other.
   c. Based on what you have come to know in this chapter, describe an example of how you might care for self and care for another Nurse under extreme conditions.

## Group Activities

- In the Chapter, you were presented with several Nursing Situations. Choose one and apply the HHE Framework.
  - Ask yourself: *How did the Nurse come to know the call for Nursing to co-create a holistic healing environment on the front lines of pandemic*?
- Which caring theory of Nursing do you see as guiding the Nurse in the Nursing Situation you chose. Why?

# Epilogue: Co-Creating a Holistic Healing Environment in Nursing Practice

*Marlaine C. Smith, RN, PhD, AHN-BC, HWNC-BC, FAAN, HSGAHN*

> *The present moment contains past and future. The secret of transformation is in the way we choose to live this very moment.*
>
> —adapted from Thich Nhat Hanh

As I was reading this book, the image of a butterfly entered my consciousness several times. The butterfly is the symbol of transformation. Perhaps it surfaced in my awareness because the authors were proposing a transformative framework for Nursing practice, one that is a shift from conventional practice, with the potential to profoundly impact the health, healing, and wellbecoming of those we serve. Those who propose transformational change must have the courage to offer a vision that challenges the status quo and the wisdom to construct a roadmap as a guide along the path to realize the vision. Drs. Shirley Gordon and Nancey France provide both. The intention to transform Nursing practice cannot be a pie-in-the-sky imagining ... it's born in the present ... in the everyday *knowingdoingbecoming* Nursing praxis as presented by Gordon and France. My purpose in writing this epilogue is to share the meaningful reflections that I had in reading the book and to recommend how the ideas presented can propel us to the transformation we are desperate to experience in Nursing education and practice.

In an analysis of 50 years of discourse related to the focus of the discipline of Nursing, four themes emerged: human wholeness; health, healing, wellbeing (wellbecoming); human-environment-health relationship; and caring (Smith, 2019). Of those, the interrelationship of environment with health, healing, and wellbeing probably remains the most neglected theme as far as knowledge development and praxis within the discipline. The events of the recent past have precipitated a sharper focus on the importance of the human-environment-health relationship. One obvious example is the COVID-19 pandemic drawing attention to the environmental threats to health and the importance of creating environments that reduce the threat of infection and support wellbeing. During the pandemic, we witnessed how the hospital environment was perceived as toxic and exploitive of Nurses and other healthcare providers, leaving in its wake many disillusioned and suffering Nurses leaving the profession. We've observed the impact of climate-generated disasters such as drought, fires, rising oceans, and more severe storms on health, and we've heard the warnings from the scientific community that a lack of action now threatens the future viability of human life as we know it. The environment of structural racism in the United States and its impact on health and wellbeing of people of color, including, but not limited to, prevalent health disparities, is another call to attend to the human-environment-health interrelationship. Yet another is how war, violence, and political divisions manifest deep wounds that impact wellbeing and cry out for action to promote peace and healing.

These are some examples of the critical human-environment-health relationships that beg for our urgent attention. But again, transformation isn't born in some future action; it happens in the present with knowing participation in change (Barrett, 2020). The word *transforming* means transcending or going beyond form ... what exists. And those engaging in transformative change don't begin by denying what exists but acknowledging it and imagining possibilities, freely choosing intentional actions consistent with it, and getting involved in creating change (Barrett, 2020). The publication of this book focusing on the holistic healing environment and how Nurses co-create it in their practice could not be more timely.

The authors of this book have charted for us an uplifting and hopeful way forward, full of power and possibilities. They ground their Holistic Healing Environment (HHE) framework within the Unitary-Transformative Paradigm (Newman, Sime, & Corcoran-Perry, 1991) and unitary caring science (Smith, 2020a; Watson, 2018; Watson & Smith, 2002) and draw from the ideas of Nightingale (1859/1969), Rogers (1992), and Watson (2018) as foundational theories that inform HHE. They make the leap that Newman, Sime, and Corcoran-Perry (1991) predicted over 30 years ago: asserting that the unitary-transformative worldview is necessary for the full expression of Nursing knowledge and practice.

Gordon and France rightly center Nursing as the professional discipline poised and prepared to take the leadership in co-creating healing environments based on its knowledge base and history. As early as women and men cared for the sick and injured in homes, convents, or monasteries, there has been attention to the need for restful, hallowed surroundings to support the healing process. Nightingale (1859/1969) formalized these practices into a conceptual framework of caring for the sick that had environment as its foreground. For Nightingale, Nursing was putting the person in the best condition for Nature to act. The activities of facilitating the best condition included attention to environmental dimensions such as: ventilation, cleanliness, air, water, noise, variety, food, and light. But Nightingale did not address a key dimension of the healing environment: the caregiver. This is the center of the healing environment for Gordon and France: Nurse as the healing environment, co-creator of sacred space to support the emergence of healing. The authors' novel definition of "Nurse" is "a cocreator of healing and peace through caring science; helps the other to find meaning in living experiences and wellbecoming; soul whisperer and healer".

Rogers (1970, 1992) introduced a unitary worldview, radical at the time of its introduction. Unitary refers to the conceptualization of human beings as irreducible human energy fields, integral and in mutual process with irreducible environmental energy fields. Both of these energy fields are identifiable by pattern, and patterning of the human-environment field happens continuously in the dynamic mutual process of change. Energy fields are pandimensional, meaning "a nonlinear domain without spatial and temporal attributes" (Rogers, 1992, p. 29)—in other words, beyond the limitations of our "usual" perceptions of three-dimensional space and linear time. Perceptions, experiences, and expressions are the manifestations of pattern (Cowling, 1997). Change is rhythmic, continuous, and fluctuating in dynamic high-low frequency wave patterns, and human beings participate knowingly in the change process including in co-creating a healing environment (Rogers, 1992).

Jean Watson (1985, 2018) adopted a unitary worldview in her later theoretical work. Her conceptualizations of unitary caring science (UCS) are a reflection of a maturing discipline (Watson, Smith,

& Cowling, 2019). The cosmology of UCS includes interconnectedness and undivided wholeness, eternal here and now, evolutionary and participatory nature of change, paradox, and love (Watson, Smith, & Cowling, 2019). The theory of unitary caring (Smith, 1999; Watson, Smith, & Cowling, 2019; Smith, 2020a), within UCS, specifies the meaning of caring within a unitary worldview in the concepts of: manifesting intentions, appreciating pattern, attuning to dynamic flow, experiencing the Infinite, and inviting creative emergence. Watson's (1985) theory of transpersonal caring and the transpersonal caring moment are imbued with images of a soul-to-soul connection between person and Nurse that transcends space, time, and physicality. This caring moment is a turning point for healing. In her construction of UCS, Watson describes the Ethic of Belonging in an infinite field of Universal Consciousness—Cosmic Love, that caring and love are the most universal, tremendous and mysterious of cosmic forces, and that love is the greatest source of healing. Finally, she states that professional unitary caring praxis integrates caring-healing modalities and the ten caritas processes (Watson, 2018, pp. 41–42).

Within the UCS view of human-environment, the Nurse is energy field integral with a larger environmental energy field and inseparable from the patient's energy field. Healing, originating from the root word *haelen,* meaning whole or possessing integrity, has been defined as "being in right relationship" (Quinn, 1989) and deepening awareness of one's unitary nature (connectedness with Self, others) (Smith, 2002) among others. Quinn makes the point that her definition is even aligned with the generic process of wound healing, a process of skin and tissues knitting together in "right relationship" with the whole. At a metaphysical level, the concept of healing is a process in which right relationship and awakening to wholeness are experienced as peace, joy, harmony, gratitude, and unconditional love. The Nurse, as co-creator of the healing environment, prepares herself to be the healing environment. This can happen in the hospital room, at a distance during a telehealth visit, in a classroom with students, in the C-Suite with healthcare leaders, or at a meeting with legislators advocating for policies addressing climate change, health equity, or gun violence. The Nurse participates in the structuring of the human-environment mutual process through knowing participation.

Gordon and France use beautiful, evocative terms to inspire our understanding of the Holistic Healing Environment (HHE) framework. They weave together a tapestry from threads of the foundational theories that they draw from, such as "wellbecoming," "energyspirit," and "integral presence" (Phillips, 2015, 2017, 2019), and coin their own terms, such as "living experience," "*knowing-doingbecoming,*" "*heartmindbodysoul,*" "soul whisperer," and "compassionate unity." The foundational concepts and those newly developed are abstract, unfamiliar terms to the reader at first exposure. All sciences have abstract, unfamiliar terms that are part of the language of the science, and unitary caring science is no exception. Those studying the science must learn the meaning of those terms. The beauty of the HHE framework is that any caring theory can be included within the tapestry of HHE concepts of patterns of knowing (Carper, 1978; Chinn & Kramer, 2018; Munhall, 1993; White, 1995; Willis & Leone-Sheehan, 2019), caring ingredients (Mayeroff, 1971), and attributes of caring (Roach, 1987/2002). All concepts are clearly defined throughout the text to facilitate comprehension and synthesis.

I opened this chapter with reflections on transformation, asserting that the ideas presented in the book can truly transform Nursing practice. The following are recommendations for how to participate knowingly in this transformation:

For Nurse educators:

1. Adopt the book and introduce the concepts early in the Nursing curriculum as one of the first books read by Nursing students. A critical error in Nursing curricula occurs when students begin their introduction to Nursing with courses in pathophysiology or health assessment, because students have no overriding framework within which they can integrate this knowledge. Nursing becomes a focus on disease, diagnosis, or problem identification. Students have difficulty grasping the distinct perspective of their discipline and the essence of their practice. An understanding of this quintessential knowledge should happen first to serve as a foundation upon which to scaffold all other knowledge. This book can ground students in the meaning of the professional discipline of Nursing. The engaging exercises within each chapter invite self-reflection and creative and critical thinking about such topics as "why I wanted to become a Nurse" or "what is my definition of 'Nurse' and 'Nursing.'" The authors have created an instructional primer within the structure of the book. For example, each chapter has objectives, clearly defined key concepts, prewriting activities and thoughtful reflections, group activities, and chapter takeaways. Moving through the book as organized assists faculty in how to engage students with this often-abstract material. As stated earlier, definitions of new terms are repeated throughout the book so that they become more familiar and integrated within the context of new material.
2. Embrace the HHE framework as a guide to structuring teaching-learning environments with students. Students learn from their experiences. When students experience the quality of a holistic healing environment with their faculty in didactic (classroom or online) or practice (clinical) courses, they can witness their faculty's way of being, and grasp the nuances related to creating a healing environment in their practice (clinical) settings.
3. Draw on the Nurses' living experiences to inspire and clarify how the HHE framework can be lived in practice. Encourage students to share their living experiences of Nursing in didactic and practice (clinical) courses in post conferences and link the elements in the story to the concepts in the framework, including the integrated Nursing theories. The shift in perspective is to place the focus on how Nursing was lived with this person (family, community), rather than focusing only on the person Nursed. This addresses what Benner and colleagues (2010) refer to as the "formation" of the Nurse.
4. Use the exemplars throughout the book as the ground for teaching Nursing. The authors have provided excellent examples of contexts with Nurses and patients. The use of the framework aids in integrating all patterns of knowing, including the empiric knowledge related to knowledge from other disciplines (pathophysiology, pharmacology, psychology, etc.); however, the ground or focus is always Nursing qua Nursing, meaning the philosophic/ theoretic knowledge of the discipline and how this is integrated into knowing/doing/becoming: Nursing praxis.

5. Design simulation scenarios that lend themselves to students practicing how to live the HHE framework. For example, they might be challenged on how to be authentically present, how to prepare self as an instrument of healing, or how to cocreate a holistic healing environment in multiple contexts.

For Nurses in practice:

6. Introduce the book in a hospital or other healthcare setting's "book/journal club." Begin by sharing personal stories of experiencing being a "soul whisperer" or "compassionate unity." Dialogue about the meaning of the concepts, including how this approach has been or can be part of their living experience as Nurses. Use the exercises in each chapter of the book to guide the dialogue.
7. Post examples of co-creating healing environments on the electronic or stationery bulletin boards or publish them in newsletters.
8. Share the stories of Nurses' living experiences of co-creating healing environments with the public in magazines, blogs, podcasts, community newsletters, newspapers, etc. so that the essence of Nursing can be better understood. Invite creative expressions such as poetry, music, dance, and visual art to express Nurses' living experiences.
9. Share the book in interprofessional practice environments to invite discussion about Nursing's unique contribution to the team and how to support the full realization of Nursing practice within interprofessional teams.
10. Develop an assessment tool to evaluate the quality of holistic healing environments in practice and a valid and reliable tool to measure the quality of a holistic healing environment for research.

Gordon and France state that their intent in writing this book is to invite those reading it "to come to know Nursing in a profound way." I believe that those reading it will indeed come to know the power and beauty of Nursing practice in a deeper way. The authors gift us with a transformative vision of Nursing praxis and the roadmap to reach it. The Holistic Healing Environment framework was developed "to guide the Nurse in concert with caring theories of Nursing in cocreating a holistic healing environment within and through caring and healing" (Gordon & France, 2022). I look forward to seeing the fruits of the authors' labors of love transforming the praxis of Nursing and ultimately the wellbecoming of those they serve.

Appendix

# Nursing Situations Kaleidoscope

| Unit | Chapter | Nursing Situation Title | Wellbecoming Concern(s) | Practice Setting | Population | Additional Populations | Key Learning Concepts |
|---|---|---|---|---|---|---|---|
| I | 1 | *"I'm Your Nurse. And I'm here with You"* | Fear<br>Human connection<br>Loss | Hospital Based COVID Unit | Adult male/ COVID19 Infection<br>CHF<br>Fever<br>Difficulty breathing | Adults in intensive care settings | Nurse as healer<br>Interdisciplinary collaboration<br>Trusting team's competence |
| | 2 | – | – | – | – | – | – |
| | 3 | *"Forever Changed"* | Anger<br>Safety<br>Connection | School health setting<br>Middle school | Young boy (7th Grade)<br>Type I Diabetes Frequent health room visits | All children and adolescents who live with chronic health conditions. | Caring for self<br>Diabetes Education<br>Importance of hydration<br>Unknowing participation<br>Knowing person as energyspirit<br>Interconnectedness<br>*alternating rhythms of perceiving-experiencing* |
| II | 4 | *"I trust you"* | Anxiety<br>Lack of focus<br>Human Connection | NP Pediatric Primary Care | Young Children/ Mothers<br>ADHD | Children experiencing anxiety: hospitals, schools, camps, etc. | Calming energy<br>Reiki<br>Presence<br>Aroma therapy<br>Trust |
| | 5 | *"Peacefulness and Calm"* | Call for peacefulness and calm | ICU | Adult Male/ adult sons | All adults in stressful, intense settings. | Reiki<br>Creating space<br>Healing<br>Nurse presence<br>Patient preference |
| | 6 | *"150 Miles an Hour"* | Stress<br>Burnout | Hospital | Nurses | Staff in all health care settings | Caring for Self<br>Peer-to-peer support<br>Caring presence<br>Alternative therapies |

| Unit | Chapter | Nursing Situation Title | Wellbecoming Concern(s) | Practice Setting | Population | Additional Populations | Key Learning Concepts |
|---|---|---|---|---|---|---|---|
| III | 7 | *"Struggling to Walk the Walk"* | Self-reflection<br>Trusting self<br>Forgiving mistakes | Hospital | Nurse/<br>gender affirmation surgery | All adults in the LGBTQ community. | Building rapport<br>Team unity<br>Mis-gendering<br>LGBTQ sensitive care |
| | 8 | *"Listen to my voice"* | Nurse Presence<br>Maintaining family presence<br>Promoting healing environment<br>Comfort | Military Hospital<br>Labor and Delivery | Adult woman<br>Labor and Delivery | All women in labor<br>Families | Take charge of the environment<br>Human connection through technology<br>Respect for person |
| | 9 | *"I am so scared I'm going to flunk out"* | Anxiety<br>Emotional trauma<br>Connection with family | BSN Program | Undergraduate Nursing Students/<br>Test Anxiety Homesickness | Young Adult Students<br>Young adults | Coming to know self<br>Holistic caring for Self<br>Co-creating a holistic healing environment in educational settings<br>Curricular designs grounded in the HHE Framework |
| | 10 | *"I'm good but I knew I wasn't"* | High Stress<br>Anxiety | Acute Care | Nurse manager | All Nurses | Deep breathing<br>Reiki<br>Caring for self<br>Coming to know self<br>Holistic Nurse Coach |
| IV | 11 | *"The Miracle of Compassionate Unity"* | Finding purpose & reason to survive | POW Camp | Nurses as POWs<br>Hunger | Nurses under extreme work environments | Caring for self<br>Nurse-to-Nurse Caring |
| | 11 | *"Let me Smell the earth"* | Getting "home"<br>Connecting with the earth<br>Connecting with God | Flight Care | Wounded Soldier (Vietnam)<br>Blindness | Veterans | Respect for person<br>Gratitude |
| | 11 | *"Goodnight Moon"* | Safety<br>Love<br>Human touch<br>Connection | War Zone | Wounded Civilian Child | Caring for persons who are different from you<br>Nurse Veterans | Trauma<br>Trust<br>Love<br>Risk<br>Overcoming hate |

| Unit | Chapter | Nursing Situation Title | Wellbecoming Concern(s) | Practice Setting | Population | Additional Populations | Key Learning Concepts |
|---|---|---|---|---|---|---|---|
| | 11 | *"Hold my hand"* | Pain<br>Human connection | During War | Wounded Soldier (Afghanistan)<br>Gunshot wound<br>Uncontrolled bleeding | Veterans<br>Families of Veterans | Emotional trauma<br>Physical trauma<br>End-of-life care<br>Nurse Presence |
| | 11 | *"Compassionate Unity"* | Healing connection<br>Safety<br>Caring for self | War Zone | Nurses<br>Wounded Soldier (Vietnam) | Nurses<br>Nurse Veterans<br>Veterans<br>Families of Veterans | Team<br>Nurse-to-Nurse caring<br>Trauma |
| | 12 | *"I'll go"* | Safety<br>Suffering<br>Pain<br>Infection<br>Nutrition | Community<br>Spanish Flu | Adults working in mines<br>Families | All community settings | Commitment<br>Contagion Holistic assessment<br>Dehydration |
| | 12 | *"The Nurses Remained"* | Safety<br>Contagion<br>Nutrition<br>Dehydration | War Zone<br>Spanish Flu | Soldiers<br>Nurses<br>WWI | Nurses<br>Nurse Veterans<br>Veterans | Nurse-to-Nurse caring<br>Gratitude |
| | 12 | *"Come up with something"* | Safety<br>Contagion | War Zone<br>Military Base<br>COVID | Soldiers<br>Nurse soldiers<br>(Afghanistan) | Nurses<br>Nurse Veterans<br>Veterans | Triage<br>Resource management<br>Entrepreneurship<br>Synergy<br>Sanitation |

# Glossary

## A

**Authentic presence**—Awareness of and coming-to-know self in synchrony and harmony within alternating rhythms guided by Mayeroff's ingredients of caring and Roach's caring attributes to choose *who I bring to practice in this moment.*

## C

**Caring circle**—Co-creating space through awareness of self within alternating rhythms to strengthen a sense of community from which emerges synchronous authentic presence.

**Caring for self**—Holistic blueprint for wholeness and self-healing through coming to know self in our wholeness and what matters most to us within our *heartmindbodysoul.*

**Centering**—An intentional process of becoming authentically present to self within *heartmindbodysoul.*

**Compassionate unity**—Emerges within integral presence and is the alternating rhythms of perceiving-experiencing *I feel you, you feel me, and I feel you feeling me* (Hübl, 2021, p. 2)—the interwoven energy field of Nurse and simultaneously the healer and healee, both healing and both being healed. Within compassionate unity, Nurse is soul whisperer and healer.

**COVID-19**—A global flu pandemic in which the first hospitalizations occurred in Wuhan, China (Senior, 2022), and quickly spread worldwide. It is the first flu pandemic in which effective vaccines were developed.

## E

**Ease**—"resonant harmony in the flow of human-environmental field patterning characterized by calm and familiar rhythms" (Smith, 2020c, p. 13).

**Energyspirit**—Replaces the concepts of person or patient and "unifies energy and spirit as a whole and transcends ideas of parts, including mind-body-spirit" (Phillips, 2017, p. 223).

**Environment**—Environment is understood as "an irreducible, pandimensional energy field identified by pattern and is integral with the human field" (Rogers, 1992, p. 29). The person-environment field includes everything external to and interacting with person (energyspirit) in a continuous mutual process.

## G

**Gender affirmation surgery**—"Provides reconstructive care that centers your vision for aligning your body and anatomy to your gender identity" (NYU Langone Health, 2022).

**Grounding**—"The process of connecting to the earth and the earth's energy field to calm the mind and focus one's inner flow of energy as a means to enhance healing endeavors" (Thornton & Mariano, 2022, p. 368); illuminates an awareness of the unity of *heartmindbodysoul.*

## H

**Healing**—Personal experience of transcending suffering; a pandimensional, nonlinear emergent mutual process of the integrality of one's *heartmindbodysoul* and environment. Nurse as soul whisperer is integrally present and in compassionate unity with other to ease and transcend suffering.

**Healing huddle**—A gathering of Nurse and staff with the intention of grounding and centering to knowingly participate as team to move through turbulence to ease for healing.

**Health**—Within the Unitary-Transformative Paradigm and HHE Framework, wellbecoming replaces the static concepts of health and wellbeing.

**Holism**—A pandimensional view of person in his/her wholeness, lifeworld, and being.

**Holistic**—Greater than and different from the sum of parts.

**Humanitarian**—A person promoting human welfare and social reform (Merriam-Webster, n.d.-a).

**Humanitarianism**—Showing concern for the welfare of humanity; being in a situation in which many human lives are in danger of harm or death (Free Dictionary, n.d.).

## I

**Ingredients of caring**—Knowing, alternating rhythms, patience, honesty, trust, humility, hope, and courage.

**Inner coherence**—The person's *heartmindbodysoul* is in harmony and synchrony.

**Nurse**—*Co-creator of healing and peace through unitary caring science; helps person to find meaning in the living experience and wellbecoming; soul whisperer, healer.*

**Integral presence**—"A perceiving-experiencing of the integrality of [persons] and the environment" (Phillips, 2015, p. 46) emerging from authentic presence, as the Nurse experiences the wholeness of self and other and the interconnectedness of self with other.

**Integrative health**—Partnering with person in his/her wholeness to support wellbecoming and find meaning in the health experience through reflection, identification of patterns, and opportunities for healing.

**Integrative healthcare**—Nurse, person, family, and interprofessional team co-coordinate conventional and complementary approaches for healing.

**Intention**—The choice to knowingly participate in the person-environment field.

## K

**Knowing participation**—The intentional mutual patterning within person and environment, which are unitary and inseparable.

***Knowingdoingbecoming***—Manifests the wholeness and alternating rhythms of healing *heartmindbodysoul.*

## L

**Living experience**—Repeating and enduring energy pattern(s) of a person's past/present/future life experience.

## M

**Moral knowing**—A pattern of knowing concerned with the development of a moral code in Nursing and determining what is morally correct.

## N

**Nurse**—Co-creator of healing and peace through unitary caring science; helps person to find meaning in the living experience and wellbecoming; soul whisperer, healer.

**Nursing**—A basic and applied science, discipline, art with its own unique, abstract, and substantive body of knowledge created from basic and applied research and development and testing of its theories; a learned profession. Persons who are educated to use Nursing knowledge (science) according to nationally regulated, defined, and monitored standards for the protection and safety of healthcare for society and its members are *Nurses.*

**Nursing praxis**—The interconnectedness of a discipline's worldview, science, theories, research, education, and practice emerging as "a synthesis of thoughtful reflection, caring, and action within theory and research-driven practice" (Hines & Gaughan, 2014, p. 26); a synchrony of knowing/doing/being (Watson, 2018, p. 21).

**Nursing profession**—Defined within praxis; "consists of persons educated in the [Nursing] discipline according to nationally regulated, defined, and monitored standards (Parse, 1999, p. 275) for the protection and safety of healthcare for society and its members.

**Nursing Situation**—The aesthetic expression of the Nurse's living experience within praxis grounded in caring science and embodies all patterns of knowing and focuses on what matters most to persons.

## P

**Pandemic**—"An outbreak of a disease that occurs over a wide geographic area (such as multiple countries or continents) and typically affects a significant proportion of the population" (Merriam-Webster, n.d.-b)

**Pandimensionality**—A "nonlinear domain without spatial or temporal attributes" (Rogers, 1992, p. 29).

**Patterns of knowing**—Are manifested as repeating/enduring waves of *knowing/doing/becoming* that are always integral, evolving, and emerging. Currently there are 11 patterns: aesthetic, emancipatory, empirical, ethical, intuitive, narrative, personal, sociopolitical, spiritual, technological, and unknowing.

**Person**—A person is understood as an energyspirit (Phillips, 2015), which is "an irreducible, indivisible, pandimensional energy field identified by pattern and manifesting characteristics that are specific to the whole and which cannot be predicted from knowledge of the parts" (Rogers, 1992, p. 29). The concepts person and energyspirit are used interchangeably throughout the book.

**Praxis**—The interconnectedness of a discipline's worldview, science, theories, research, education, and practice emerging as "a synthesis of thoughtful reflection, caring, and action within theory and research-driven practice" (Hines & Gaughan, 2014, p. 26); a synchrony of knowing/doing/being (Watson, 2018, p. 21).

## R

**Reiki**—Is "spiritually guided life energy" (New York Presbyterian Hospital, 2022, par. 4) connecting us with our environment. As an energy therapy, persons may experience relaxation, peacefulness, calmness, and wellbecoming. Reiki therapy can involve touch or no touch.

**Resilience**—"The *capacity to prepare* for, recover from and adapt in the face of stress, adversity, trauma, or tragedy" (HeartMath® Institute, 2021a, para 3 ln 1–2).

## S

**Self-care**—Focuses on strategies to address our deficits and weaknesses; often grounded in feeling guilty or being upset with ourselves. A focus on strategies provides a piece-by-piece plan trying to balance everything to fix us.

**Self-made Nurses**—Persons (primarily women) portrayed as humanitarians easing the suffering of soldiers, protecting their dignity, and preserving their humanity.

**Soul Whisperer**—Nurse interconnects with person soul-to-soul through "pandimensional thoughts such as soothing, tender, quieting, and loving, giving illumination and radiance" (Phillips, 2015, p. 46) to transcend suffering.

**Spanish Flu**—A global flu pandemic that started as a localized outbreak in a U.S. Army camp in Kansas and spread within days to New York City and then worldwide (Centers for Disease Control and Prevention, 2019).

## T

**Trauma**—"The subjective experience of an event, or series of events, that overwhelms an individual's capacity to cope" (HeartMath® Institute, 2021b, p. 1).

**Transgender**—"Designating a person whose sense of personal identity and gender does not correspond to that person's sex at birth, or which does not otherwise conform to conventional notions of sex and gender" (Simpson, Weiner, & Oxford University Press, 1988).

**Turbulence ease**—"Shifting patterning of turbulence to ease" (Smith, 2020c, p. 18). The Nurse as environmental field integrally present with other can shift the patterning of turbulence to ease.

## U

**Unknowing**—Choosing to be open in *heartmindbodysoul* to come to know other in the moment.

**Unknowing participation**—Lack of awareness and attention to mutual patterning within person and environment, often manifested within a task-oriented practice approach.

## W

**War** (noun)—Hostile contention by means of armed forces, carried on between nations, states, or rulers, or between parties in the same nation or state; the employment of armed forces against a foreign power, or against an opposing party in the state (Simpson & Weiner, 1988).

**Wellbecoming**—A process through which one knowingly participates in changing patterns and manifestations of wholeness and healing.

**Wholeness**—*Heartmindbodysoul.*

# References


Alexander, K. L. (n.d.). *Aileen Cole Stewart.* National Women's History Museum. https://www.womenshistory.org/education-resources/biographies/aileen-cole-stewart

Alltucker, K. (December 20, 2021). Hospitals prepare for omicron even as Nurses exit. *USA Today,* 3A.

American Nurses Association. (n.d.). *What is nursing?* https://www.nursingworld.org/practice-policy/workforce/what-is-nursing/

American Red Cross. (n.d.-a). *Founder Clara Barton.* https://www.redcross.org/content/dam/redcross/enterprise-assets/about-us/history/history-clara-barton-v5.pdf

American Red Cross. (n.d.-b). *Jane Delano: Founder of the American Red Cross Nursing Service.* https://www.redcross.org/content/dam/redcross/enterprise-assets/about-us/history/nursing-history-jane-delano.pdf

Andrews, C. (2013, October 14). *Crimea—The first modern war. E&T: Engineering and Technology.* https://eandt.theiet.org/content/articles/2013/10/crimea-the-first-modern-war/

Andrews, E. (2020, April 23). *8 facts about the Crimean War.* https://www.history.com/news/8-things-you-may-not-know-about-the-crimean-war

Arlington National Cemetery. (n.d.). *Spanish-American War Nurses Memorial.* https://www.arlingtoncemetery.mil/Explore/Monuments-and-Memorials/Spanish-American-War-Nurses

Army Nurse Corps Association. (n.d.). *Contributions of the U.S. Army Nurse Corps in World War I.* https://e-anca.org/History/Topics-in-ANC-History/Contributions-of-the-US-Army-Nurse-Corps-in-WWI

Barrett, E. A. M. (2020). Elizabeth Barrett's theory of knowing participation in change. In M. C. Smith (Ed.), *Nursing theories and nursing practice* (pp. 479–491). F. A. Davis.

Barry, C. D., Gordon, S. C., & King, B. M. (2015). *Nursing case studies in caring: Across the practice spectrum.* Springer.

Benner, P., Sutphen, M., Leonard, V., & Day, L. (2010). *Educating nurses: A call for radical transformation.* Jossey Bass.

Biography.com Editors. (2021, August 11). *Biography: Harriet Tubman.* https://www.biography.com/activist/harriet-tubman

Bollinger, R., & Ray, S. (2021). COVID omicron variant: What you need to know. *Johns Hopkins Medicine,* https://www.hopkinsmedicine.org/health/conditions-and-diseases/coronavirus/covid-omicron-variant-what-you-need-to-know

Bollinger, R., Ray, S., & Maragakis, L. (2022). COVID variants: What you should know. *Johns Hopkins Medicine,* https://www.hopkinsmedicine.org/health/conditions-and-diseases/coronavirus/a-new-strain-of-coronavirus-what-you-should-know

Boykin, A., & Schoenhofer, S. (2001). *Nursing as caring: A model for transforming practice.* Jones and Bartlett Publishers and National League for Nursing.

Bradley-Sanders, C. (n.d.). *Bellevue School of Nursing. The Lillian and Clarence De La Chapelle Medical Archives.* https://archives.med.nyu.edu/collections/bellevue-school-of-nursing

Brathovde, A. (2017). Teaching nurses Reiki energy therapy for self-care. *International Journal for Human Caring, 21*(1), 20–25.

Britannica, The Editors of Encyclopaedia. (2021, August 20). *Clara Maass.* https://www.britannica.com/biography/Clara-Maass

Britannica, The Editors of Encyclopaedia. (2022, May 20). *Jane A. Delano.* https://www.britannica.com/biography/Jane-A-Delano

Britt, K.C., Scholar, J., & Acton, G. (2022). Exploring the meaning of spirituality and spiritual care with help from Viktor Frankl. *Journal of Holistic Nursing, 40*(1), 46–55.

Burrows, L. M. (2020, August 19). *Mama Josie and the angels of Bataan.* https://lynettemburrows.com/mama-josie-and-the-angels-of-bataan/

Butcher, H. (2021). Principles of integrality, resonancy, and helicy. In H. Butcher (Ed.), *The Science of Unitary Human Beings 2.0.* https://pressbooks.uiowa.edu/rogeriannursingscience/chapter/chapter-5-introduction-to-the-principles/

Butcher, H. K., & Malinski, V. M. (2020). Martha E. Rogers' science of unitary human beings. In M. C. Smith (Ed.) *Nursing theories and nursing practice* (5th ed., pp. 237–257). F. A. Davis Co.

Carper, B. A. (1978). Fundamental patterns of knowing in nursing. *Advances in Nursing Science, 1*(1), 13–24.

Centers for Disease Control and Prevention. (2019, March 20) *1918 pandemic (H1N1 virus).* https://www.cdc.gov/flu/pandemic-resources/1918-pandemic-h1n1.html

Childs, J. W. (2021). How long did it take to develop the flu vaccine? *The Weather Channel.* https://weather.com/health/news/2021-01-21-how-long-did-it-take-to-develop-the-flu-shot

Chinn, P. L., & Kramer, M. K. (2018). *Knowledge development in nursing: Theory and process* (10th ed.). Elsevier.

Clara Barton Birthplace Museum. (2017). *Clara's life.* https://www.clarabartonbirthplace.org/claras-life/

Cody, W. K. (1995). About all those paradigms: Many in the university, two in nursing. *Nursing Science Quarterly, 8*(4), 144–147.

Cogan, R., & Smilios, M. (2020). #5 of 52 nurse profiles: Aileen Cole Stewart. *American Nurse.* https://www.myamerican-nurse.com/5-of-52-nurse-profiles-aileen-cole-stewart/

College of Physicians of Philadelphia. (2018). *History of Vaccines:Influenza.* https://www.historyofvaccines.org/content/articles/influenza

Cowling, W. R. (1997). Pattern appreciation: The unitary science/practice of reaching for essence. In M. Madrid (Ed.), *Patterns of Rogerian knowing* (pp. 129–142). National League for Nursing Press.

Dossey, B. M., & Luck, S. (2015). Nurse coaching and leadership. In B. M. Dossey, S. Luck, & B. G. Schaub (Eds.). *Nurse coaching: Integrative approaches for health and wellbeing* (pp. 387–404). International Nurse Coach Association.

Duchscher, J. B. (2008). A process of becoming: The stages of new nursing graduate professional role transition. *Journal of Continuing Education in Nursing, 39*(10), 441–450.

Dunphy, L. M. H. (2020). Florence Nightingale's conceptualizations of nursing. In M. C. Smith (Ed.), *Nursing theories and nursing practice* (5th ed., pp. 35–54). F. A. Davis Co.

Duquesne University School of Nursing. (n.d.). *The history of wartime nurses.* https://onlinenursing.duq.edu/history-wartime-nurses/

Encyclopedia.com. (2019). *Schuyler, Louisa Lee (1837–1926).* https://www.encyclopedia.com/women/encyclopedias-almanacs-transcripts-and-maps/schuyler-louisa-lee-1837-1926

Fee, E. & Garofalo, M.E. (2010). Florence Nightingale and the Crimean war. *American Journal of Public Health, 100*(9), 1591.

Fleck, D. (1995). *The handbook of humanitarian law in armed conflicts.* Oxford University Press.

France, N.E.M. (1994). Unitary human football players. In M. Madrid and E. Barrett (Eds.) *Rogers' scientific art of nursing practice* (p. 197–206). New York: National League for Nursing Press ISBN 0-88737-608-8.

France, N, & Gordon, S.C. Caring for Self: Nurturing Wholeness and Well-Being Webinar (2020, June 18th). Cross Country Health Care and Florida Atlantic University College of Nursing.

Free Dictionary. (n.d.). Humanitarianism. *Free Dictionary.* https://www.thefreedictionary.com/humanitarianism

Goldenberg, G. 1992. *Nurses of a different stripe: A history of the Columbia University School of Nursing 1892–1992.* Columbia University School of Nursing.

Graduate Nurses in the Spanish-American War. (n.d.). [Unpublished pdf]

Greenspan, J. (2019, October 28). *The charge of the light brigade, 160 years ago. History.* https://www.history.com/news/the-charge-of-the-light-brigade-160-years-ago

Haley, M. (2013, December). *United States Sanitatary Commission records. Women's Central Association of Relief records, 1861–1866. New York Public Library Archives & Manuscripts.* https://archives.nypl.org/mss/22266

HeartMath® Institute. (2021a). *Resilience and the emotional landscape.* https://www.heartmath.org/resources/downloads/resilience-and-the-emotional-landscape/

HeartMath® Institute. (2021b). *The Resilient Heart.* https://www.heartmath.org/training/trauma-sensitive-certification/

Hektor, L. M. (1994a). Part I: Childhood and early education (1914–1937). In V. M. Malinski & E. A. M. Barrett (Eds.). *Martha E. Rogers: Her life and her work* (pp. 10–14). F. A. Davis Co.

Hektor, L. M. (1994b). Part II: Years of work and study (1938–1953). In V. M. Malinski & E. A. M. Barrett (Eds.). *Martha E. Rogers: Her life and her work* (pp. 15–18) F. A. Davis Co.

Higgins, L.P. (1996). Army nurses in wartime: Distinction and pride. *Military Medicine, 161*(8), 472.

Hines, M. E., & Gaughan, J. (2014). Pediatric nurses acknowledging praxis: Recognizing caring in reflective narratives. *International Journal for Human Caring, 18*(3), 26–35.

History.com Editors (2003). War in Iraq begins. https://www.history.com/this-day-in-history/war-in-iraq-begins

Hübl, T. (2021). Resilience is through relation. In *The Collective Experience of Trauma and Healing*. The HeartMath® Institute, 45.1, p. 2. https://www.heartmath.org/training/trauma-sensitive-certification/

*It happened here: Anna Maxwell*. (n.d.). New York-Presbyterian https://healthmatters.nyp.org/it-happened-here-anna-maxwell/

Jones, M. M. (n.d.). *American experience: American nurses in World War I. PBS*. https://www.pbs.org/wgbh/americanexperience/features/the-great-war-american-nurses-world-war-1/

Kagan, P. N., Smith, M. C., Cowling, W. R., & Chinn, P. L. (2009). A nursing manifesto: An emancipatory call for knowledge development, conscience, and praxis. *Nursing Philosophy, 11(1)*, 67–84.

Lim-Saco, F., Kilat, C. M., & Locsin, R. (2018). Synchronicity in human–space–time: A theory of nursing engagement in a global community. *International Journal for Human Caring, 22*(1), 1–10. https://connect.springerpub.com/content/sgrijhc%3A%3A%3A22%3A%3A%3A1%3A%3A%3A29.full.pdf

MacLean, M. (n.d.). *Clara Barton (The angel of the battlefield). Ehistory: Ohio State University Department of History*. https://ehistory.osu.edu/biographies/clara-barton-angel-battlefield#:~:text=There%20she%20worked%20as%20a,that%20of%20the%20male%20clerks

Malinski, M. (1994). A family of strong-willed women. In V.M. Malinski & E.A.M. Barrett (Eds.). *Martha Rogers: Her life and her work*. F.A. Davis Company.

Maragakis, L. (2021). Coronavirus second wave, third wave and beyond: What causes a COVID surge. *Johns Hopkins Medicine*, https://www.hopkinsmedicine.org/health/conditions-and-diseases/coronavirus/first-and-second-waves-of-coronavirus

Mayeroff, M. (1971). *On caring*. Harper & Row.

McCraty, R., Atkinson, M., & Bradley, R. T. (2004). Electrophysiological evidence of intuition: Part 1. The surprising role of the heart. *Journal of Alternative and Complementary Medicine, 10*(1), 133–143.

McDonald, L. (2013). The timeless wisdom of Florence Nightingale. *Canadian Nurse, 109*(2), 36.

Merriam-Webster. (n.d.-a). Humanitarian. *Merriam-Webster dictionary*. https://www.merriam-webster.com/dictionary/humanitarian

Merriam-Webster. (n.d.-b). Pandemic. *Merriam-Webster* dictionary. *https://www.merriam-webster.com/dictionary/pandemic*

Morphet, J., Griffiths, D., Beattie, J., & Innes, K. (2019). Managers' experiences of prevention and management of workplace violence against health care staff: A descriptive exploratory study. *Journal of Nursing Management, 27*(4), 781–791. https://doi.org/10.1111/jonm.12761

Munhall P. L. (1993). "Unknowing": Toward another pattern of knowing in nursing. *Nursing Outlook 41*(3), 125–128.

National Women's History Museum. (2019, July 8). *African American nurses in World War II*. https://www.womenshistory.org/articles/african-american-nurses-world-war-ii

National WWII Museum. (2021, May 5). *Nurse POWs: Angels of Bataan and Corregidor*. https://www.nationalww2museum.org/war/articles/nurse-pows-bataan-and-corregidor

NDTV. (2021, August 31). *Last US soldier leaves Afghanistan, ending America's longest war*. https://www.ndtv.com/world-news/last-us-troops-leave-afghanistan-ending-20-year-war-pentagon-2524242

Newman, M. A., Sime, A. M., & Corcoran-Perry, S. A. (1991). The focus of the discipline of nursing. *Advances in Nursing Science, 14*(1), 1–6.

New York Presbyterian Hospital. (2022). *The healing energy of Reiki and the mind-body connection*. https://www.nyp.org/patients-and-visitors/advances-consumers/issues/the-healing-energy-of-reiki-and-the-mind-body-connection

New York State Nurses Association. (n.d.). *First nurse and abolitionist icon to grace $20 bill*. https://www.nysna.org/first-nurse-and-abolitionist-icon-grace-20-bill#.YX1zDJ7MJnJ

Nightingale, F. (1859/1969). *Notes on Nursing: What it is and what it is not*. Lippincott.

NYU Langone Health. (2022). Transgender surgery services. https://nyulangone.org/locations/plastic-surgery/transgender-surgery-services

Parse, R. P. (1999). Nursing: The discipline and the profession. *Nursing Science Quarterly, 12*(4), 275–276.

Phillips, J. R. (2015). Martha E. Rogers: Heretic and heroine. *Nursing Science Quarterly, 28*(1), 42–48.

Phillips, J. R. (2017). New Rogerian theoretical thinking about unitary science. *Nursing Science Quarterly, 30*(3), 223–226. doi.org/10.1177/0894318417708411

Phillips, J. (2019). Unitariology and the changing frontiers of the science of unitary human beings. *Nursing Science Quarterly, 32*(3), 207–213.

Quinn, J. F. (1989). On healing, wholeness, and the haelen effect. *Nursing and Health Care, 10*(10), 552–556.

Quinn, J. F. (2017). And then a miracle occurs. *Explore, 13*(4), 268–269.

Quinn, J. F. (2022). Transpersonal human caring and healing. In M. A. B. Helming, D. A. Shields, K. M. Avino, & W. E. Rosa (Eds.). *Dossey & Keegan's holistic nursing: A handbook for practice* (8th ed., pp. 97–106). Jones & Bartlett Learning.

Riegel, F., Crossetti, M. D. G. O., Martini, J. G., & Nes, A. A. G. (2021). Florence Nightingale's theory and her contributions to holistic critical thinking in nursing. *Revista Brasileira de Enfermagem, 74*(2), 1–5. https://doi.org/10.1590/0034-7167-2020-0139

Roach, M. S. (2002). *Caring, the human mode of being. A blueprint for the health professions* (2nd rev. ed.). Canadian Hospital Association Press.

Roach, S. (1987). *The human act of caring.* Canadian Hospital Association.

Rogers, M. E. (1970). *An introduction to the theoretical basis of Nursing.* F. A. Davis Co.

Rogers, M. E. (1988). Nursing science and art: A prospective. *Nursing Science Quarterly, 1*(3), 99–102.

Rogers, M.E. (1990). Nursing: Science of unitary, irreducible, human beings: Update 1990. In E.A.M. Barrett (Ed.). *Visions of Rogers' science-based nursing,* p. 5–11. National League for Nursing.

Rogers, M. E. (1992). Nursing science and the space age. *Nursing Science Quarterly, 5*(1), 27–34.

Saad, L. (2022, January 12). *Military brass, judges among professions at new image lows.* GALLUP. https://news.gallup.com/poll/388649/military-brass-judges-among-professions-new-image-lows.aspx

Sandelowski, M. (1991). Telling stories: Narrative approaches in qualitative research. *Image: Journal of Nursing Scholarship, 23*(3), 161–166.

Senior, R. (2022). Similarities between Spanish Flu and the COVID-19 pandemic. *American Nurse.* https://www.myamericannurse.com/similarities-between-spanish-flu-and-the-covid-19-pandemic/

Simpson, J. A., Weiner, E. S. C., & Oxford University Press. (1988). *The Oxford English Dictionary.* Clarendon Press.

Singleton, M. (2019, November 8). *Flashback Friday—Harriet Tubman's overlooked story as a nurse. UVA School of Nursing.* https://www.nursing.virginia.edu/news/flashback-harriet-tubman-nurse/

Smith, M. C. (1999). Caring and the science of unitary human beings. *Advances in Nursing Science, 21*(4), 14–28.

Smith, M. C. (2002). Health, healing, and the myth of the hero journey. *Advances in Nursing Science, 24*(4), 1–13.

Smith, M. C. (2019). Regenerating Nursing's disciplinary purpose. *Advances in Nursing Science, 42*(1), 3–16.

Smith, M. C. (2020a). Marlaine Smith's theory of unitary caring. In M. C. Smith (Ed.), *Nursing theories and nursing practice* (5th ed., pp. 493–502). F. A. Davis Co.

Smith, M.D. (2020b). *Nursing theories and nursing practice* (5th ed.). F.A. Davis Co.

Smith, M. C. (2020c). Turbulence-ease in the rhythmic flow of patterning. *Visions: The Journal of Rogerian Nursing Science, 26*(2): 1–27.

Smith, M.C. & Parker, M. (2020). Nursing theory and the discipline of nursing. In M.C. Smith (Ed.) *Nursing theories and nursing practice* (5th ed.). p. 3–16. F.A. Davis.

Smith, M. C., Zahourek, R., Hines, M. E., Engebretson, J., Wardell, D. W. (2013). Holistic nurses' stories of personal healing. *Journal of Holistic Nursing, 31*(3), 173–187.

Society of Rogerian Scholars. (n.d.-a). *Nursing according to Martha.* https://www.societyofrogerianscholars.org/definition-of-nursing

Spader, C. (2021). Nurse heroes of the pandemic. *American Nurse.* https://www.myamericannurse.com/nurse-heroes-of-the-pandemic/

Stevenson, S. S. (1976). *Lamp for a soldier: The caring story of a nurse in World War I.* North Dakota State Nurses' Association.

Stewart, A. C. (1963). Ready to serve. *American Journal of Nursing, 63*(9), 85–87. doi:10.2307/3452837

Thornton, L., & Mariano, C. (2022). Evolving from therapeutic to holistic communication. In M. A. B. Helming, D. A. Shields, K. M. Avino, & W. E. Rosa (Eds.). *Dossey & Keegan's holistic nursing: A handbook for practice* (8th ed., pp. 363–376).

Tinsley, C. & France, N.E.M. (2004). The trajectory of the Registered Nurse's exodus from the profession: A phenomenological study of the lived experience of oppression. *The International Journal for Human Caring, 8*(1), 8–12.

University of Colorado Anschutz Medical Campus. (2013). *Former CU College of Nursing Dean Jean Watson honored as "Living Legend."* https://nursing.cuanschutz.edu/about/news-archives/article/CU-nursing/former-cu-college-of-nursing-dean-jean-watson-honored-as-living-legend

U.S. Army Center of Military History. (2003, October 3). *The Army Nurse Corp* (CHM Pub 72-14). https://history.army.mil/books/wwii/72-14/72-14.htm

U.S. Bureau of Labor Statistics. (2020, April 8). *Workplace violence in healthcare, 2018.* https://www.bls.gov/iif/oshwc/cfoi/workplace-violence-healthcare-2018.htm

U.S. Department of Veterans Affairs. (2011, April). *Military health history pocket card—Vietnam.* https://www.va.gov/oaa/pocketcard/m-vietnam.asp

U.S. Food & Drug Administration. (2021a). *FDA approves first COVID-19 vaccine.* https://www.fda.gov/news-events/press-announcements/fda-approves-first-covid-19-vaccine

U.S. Food & Drug Administration. (2021b, October 29). FDA authorizes Pfizer-BioNTech COVID-19 vaccine for emergency use in children 5 through 11 years of age. https://www.fda.gov/news-events/press-announcements/fda-authorizes-pfizer-biontech-covid-19-vaccine-emergency-use-children-5-through-11-years-age

VCU Libraries Social Welfare History Project. (n.d.). *Schuyler, Louisa Lee.* https://socialwelfare.library.vcu.edu/organizations/state-institutions/schuyler-louisa-lee/

Washington, D.C. (n.d.). *Vietnam Women's Memorial.* https://washington.org/find-dc-listings/vietnam-womens-memorial

Watson Caring Science Institute. (2017, October 16). Jean Watson's life journey [Video]. https://vimeo.com/238401597

Watson Caring Science Institute. (2021a). *Jean Watson—Personal profile.* https://www.watsoncaringscience.org/jean-bio/personal-profile/

Watson Caring Science Institute. (2021b). *Unitary caring science.* https://www.watsoncaringscience.org/jean-bio/caring-science-theory/

Watson, J. (1985). *Nursing: Human science and human care: A theory of nursing.* Appleton-Century Crofts.

Watson, J. (2018). *Unitary caring science: The philosophy and praxis of nursing.* University Press of Colorado.

Watson, J. (2020). Jean Watson's theory of unitary caring science and theory of human caring. In M. C. Smith (Ed.), *Nursing theories and nursing practice* (5th ed., pp. 311–331). F. A. Davis Co.

Watson, J., Malkin, G. & Alvarez, D. (2014, September 25). The caring moment. [Video] YouTube. https://www.youtube.com/watch?v=w8ajEzWfQgE).

Watson, J., & Smith, M. C. (2002). Caring science and the science of unitary human beings: A trans-theoretical discourse for nursing knowledge development. *Journal of Advanced Nursing, 37*(5), 452–461. https://doi.org/10.1046/j.1365-2648.2002.02112.x

Watson, J., Smith, M. C., & Cowling, W. R. (2019). Unitary caring science: Disciplinary evolution of nursing. In W. Rosa, J. Watson, & S. Horton-Deutsch (eds.), *A handbook for caring science* (pp. 21–36). Springer.

White, J. (1995). Patterns of knowing: Review, critique, and update. *Advances in Nursing Science, 17*(4), 73–86.

Willis, D. G., & Leone-Sheehan, D. M. (2019). Spiritual knowing: Another pattern of knowing in the discipline. *Advances in Nursing Science, 42*(1), 58–68.

# Index

www.ingramcontent.com/pod-product-compliance
Ingram Content Group UK Ltd.
Pitfield, Milton Keynes, MK11 3LW, UK
UKHW050141280726
14058UKWH00006B/766